Journey Back to the Soul

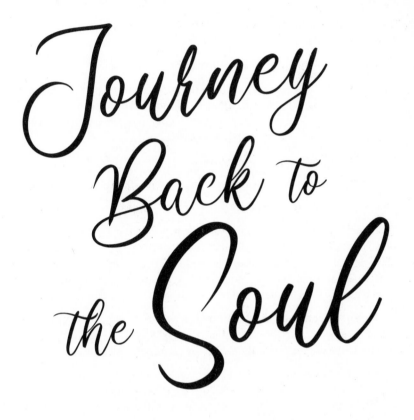

Journey Back to the Soul

CHOOSING FAITH OVER FEAR

Memarie Gayle

BRIDGE LOGOS

Newberry, FL 32669

Bridge-Logos

Newberry, FL 32669

Journey Back to the Soul: Choosing Faith over Fear
by Memarie Gayle Jobe

Printed in the United States of America.

Library of Congress Catalog Card Number: 2019953705

International Standard Book Number: 978-1-61036-218-4

Cover/Interior design by Kent Jensen | knail.com
Cover photo: Neill Jobe

Literary Agent and Editor,
L. Edward Hazelbaker
E-mail: l.edward@thewornkeyboard.com

DEDICATION

To my late father, Jerry Cupit, who taught me I could do anything I wanted in life. I just had to be willing to work hard for it.

ACKNOWLEDGMENTS

First and foremost, I thank God for chasing me down, for never giving up on me, and for blessing me in so many ways.

I thank my friends and family for always supporting me in all my creative endeavors and giving me strength to follow my dreams.

To my close friends, you have seen me at my worst and at my best. Thank you for loving me through it all and giving me a shoulder to cry on when I needed it.

To my extended family—Hazel, Ron, Jimmy, Cheri, Deana, Jon, Madison, Nelson, Nanny, and the rest of the family—thank you for lovingly welcoming me with open arms. I love you so much, and I am blessed to have you in my life!

Thank you to my church family for the Spirit-filled prayers that have lifted me to healing—both emotionally and physically. Thank you, Pastor Davis and Pastor Galen, for your leadership and for your lifetime dedication to serve. I am inspired by both of you to grow in my faith day by day.

And I give a special shout-out to Mama Gail and Pastor Sandy. You are wonderful examples of godly women to me, and I cherish you both. I now know what it truly means to have a church *family.* Sometimes in life you don't realize what you were missing until you have it.

To my dad, who is already in heaven—where I will someday see him again—thank you Daddy for always being my protector.

I knew I was always safe when you were around. I remember as a child seeing you walking around to all the doors in our house to check the locks before you tucked me in every night. And I remember you coming to my room to console me if I woke up after a bad dream. You taught me so much about music, and we made some wonderful memories that will live on forever. I love you.

Thank you, Mom, for always being my supporter and cheering me on in whatever I was doing. I remember as a child staring up at you and thinking, "I have the most beautiful mama ever!" You had me at a very young age, and I'm sure it wasn't easy, but you were a great mama. It has been a joy to have you helping me in my jewelry business and ministry over the last few years and sharing the journey with you. It has also been a joy to see you become a grandma for the first time to JD. He loves his Nana! We have so many more great memories to make. I love you Mom!

To my Granny Mary, who has always exemplified what a godly woman is, you have taught me so much through your wisdom. Your musical talents are abundant, and I am blessed to have some of that passed down to me. I will always remember my time as a little girl staying at your house and having such a great time with you. Oh, as far as I'm concerned, nobody cooks better than Granny Mary!

To Papaw Bud Gaulden, thank you for always being a kind and loving grandpa. We had some great times together growing up. Riding the tractor, riding your horses, checking on the cows, and jumping on the hay in the barn—I loved spending time with my papaw.

To Mamaw Inez, Papaw Bud Cupit, Granny Ashley, Mamaw and Papaw Garner, and all my other family members who have gone on to be with Jesus, I had the best grandparents any little girl could have asked for! I miss you all, and I love you so much! I look forward to seeing you all again one day.

Aunt Glenda, Aunt Charlotte, all my cousins, and the entire rest of my family, it would take up all the pages of this book to list you all, but you are my rock. I love you with all my heart!

—Memarie Gayle

FOREWORD

We all have a need in life to know we are not alone. And in the most difficult and challenging seasons of life, when circumstances are overwhelming, when our hearts are breaking, and when our heads are spinning trying to make sense of the senseless, we all reach out for comfort, health, and help.

The lack of those things causes pain. Some people want to medicate that pain, but the medication always wears off. Others choose to party and create their own illusions that their problems are going to cease to exist. But not so surprisingly, though their pain may be covered up for a while, sooner or later it returns.

Empathy is a tremendous healer, and there is no way you can read this book by Memarie Gayle Jobe without finding and being affected by a person who has experienced unexpected pain, shame, and guilt—who can relate to others experiencing such things, and who has yet still made a way to move forward.

I had the incredible opportunity as Memarie's pastor to have a ring-side seat through the last few years. I didn't know her well; she was just a lady singing on our platform. But I was informed that she had been diagnosed with cancer and was pressing forward.

I began to observe her countenance and determination. Week after week, and month after month, whether her hair fell out or she felt bad, she displayed a raw sense of strength, guts, grit, and determination that flowed from her heart of faith and an attitude of overcoming.

As I got to know Memarie and her husband, Neill, I found a loving couple who modeled love, quietness, joy, and compassion. So much of what I read in Memarie Gayle's book was a shock to me, because I had no idea of her journey. But I now know I have observed a champion who refuses to allow her past control either her present or her future.

This book was not just written to tell her story. It was written to encourage you to not give up and to write the story of your own journey. Regardless of where you are going in life, *Journey Back to the Soul* will inspire you to rise up, trust God, and never ever quit.

—Maury Davis,
Coach and Consultant, Maury Davis Ministries,
Global Pastor, Cornerstone Nashville

TABLE OF CONTENTS

INTRODUCTION

Writing a book was something I thought about for years. It was always in the back of my mind whispering to me. I would push it away and tell myself I would write it one day when I wasn't so busy, or maybe in my retirement years, and so forth. After all, I had never taken any writing classes in college, so I thought maybe one day I would take at least one before I wrote a book.

Of course as with most things in life, plans get altered, and life tends to go forward with or without you. One thing I have learned over the years—if you want to do something in this life, you've just got to go for it. If you are waiting on the perfect timing or the arrival of perfected abilities, you will never get anything done. Perfection is overrated anyway!

There are reasons for every event in our lives. They teach us things about ourselves and about who we are in Christ. We can find that nothing is ever in vain as long as we see the challenges in life as opportunities to grow—and then take advantage of them.

If experiences don't challenge you, they won't change you.

God will take all things and use them for good, according to His purpose.[1] And we will learn from that—if we are willing to attune ourselves to His work and follow Him.

---

1   "And we know that in all things God works for the good of those who love him, who have been called according to his purpose" (Romans 8:28).

My advice to you:

In order to fully experience and benefit from His work, you must completely give your life over to God. And doing that requires much faith, study of the Word, and prayer to fight against the fear the world pushes into us.

When our experiences challenge us, we must *choose faith over fear.*

Choosing faith over fear has been an ongoing theme in my life for as long as I can remember, but it was not until a few years ago when it was really brought to light. I let fear control me for most of my life. But once I consciously decided to choose faith over fear, my spirit became more aligned with my creator, and I became more balanced, focused, peaceful, purposeful, and joyful.

You could consider this book somewhat of a memoir, but I consider it more of a *journey back to the soul.* Throughout our lives, we evolve and grow. Sometimes we find ourselves in a place where we've gained more knowledge but in the process lost our innocence or wonder of life. We become too focused on a future moment in time, and we lose sight of the lessons and the beautiful journey along the way.

We need to learn that the journey is at times more important than where we are headed. The stringing together of all the *ah-ha* moments and hard lessons in life make up one's *soul-life.* If we are willing to truly let our wonderful creator lead us on our journeys, our lives will be filled with wonder, with surprises, with adventure, and yes, with peace.

Throughout my life's journey, I have found that God can bring me overflowing peace that's beyond understanding—even in the most difficult times.

Finally getting to the writing of this book is a good example of me pushing away fear and simply obeying God. The Holy Spirit kept whispering to me about writing my story. So here I am—surrendering, casting out fear, and moving forward in faith.

There is beauty to come from our ashes, and our victory is our testimony.

My prayer is that through my story you will see a glimpse of your own, and it will be a source of encouragement and inspiration for you in your own life's journey back to the soul.

—Memarie Gayle

CHAPTER 1

Louisiana Love Child

I grew up in the small village of Baskin, Louisiana. Yes, village—it's actually too small to be considered a town. I am an only child, so I guess you could say I became accustomed to being alone at a young age. I often played and had sleepovers with my cousins, but being an only child, I had to entertain myself on most days.

I always felt loved by my parents, grandparents, and other family; so all in all, it was a good childhood. And like most of us, the memories of my childhood consist of a vast array of flashes.

I see swinging on an old tire swing as my goat, Myrtle, pushed it with her horns. Then there's playing with my German Shepard, JJ, playing basketball with Daddy, climbing in the treehouse he built, playing with Barbie dolls with Mama, wrestling and playing Yahoo with Papaw Bud, and playing scrabble with Granny Ashley.

I remember hanging out with Mamaw Inez, singing through my magnolia-bud microphone at Mamaw and Papaw Garners, singing while Granny Mary played piano, and doing many other numerous things. One advantage to being an only child is that the cultivation of creativity inside me had room to blossom.

Since most of my playtime was spent alone, I became my own entertainment. Writing and acting out plays, writing and memorizing songs, and pretending I was on stage singing my heart out in front of thousands of people were all integral parts of my childhood. My creative world was a place where I found comfort.

Although I was happy, I do remember being a very fearful child, which I believe now was also due at least in part to being highly creative. If I accidently saw anything remotely scary on TV, it would always come back to mind when I went to bed. I had nightmares all the time, and my dad would have to come into my room and stay until I fell back to sleep.

I was so scared at times that I would lie in bed with my head under the covers for hours trying to be so quiet that I would barely breath. My mind would run wild and conjure up all kinds of things that might be going on outside my covers. If I could go back and talk to myself as a child, I would assure little Memarie that there is no reason to be afraid.

As a child of God, I know now that there is nothing to fear.

For as long as I can remember, my greatest joy came from music. There was no fear attached to music for me. I could sing in front of anyone at any time, and my parents encouraged it. Music was a constant friend to me.

My parents had their own band when I was growing up, and I loved listening and watching them rehearse every week in our home. Eventually, they let me get on stage with them when I was around nine years old, and I was completely hooked from that day forward. My mom even sewed for me my own outfit to match the rest of the band.

One stage outfit consisted of a faux suede vest trimmed in fur, and the other stage outfit was an all-black pants ensemble trimmed in silver sequins. I thought I was something else—died and gone to country cowgirl heaven! I was sooo excited! From my first time on stage, I knew I was home. I loved it! I knew what I wanted to do with my life.

Music was my first love, and I dreamed of nothing else. I watched the movie, *Coal Miner's Daughter*, the story of Loretta Lynn, at least twenty times throughout my childhood. I saw myself in Loretta Lynn, and her story gave me hope and inspiration. Like her, I was just a poor country girl who loved to sing and entertain. I dreamed of making records and touring all over the country. To me, that sounded like heaven on earth!

I was saved and baptized at nine years old, but we were not what you would call involved church members. As a matter of fact, Daddy stopped going to church altogether at one point. A deacon at the church constantly judged and condemned him for playing music at venues where alcohol was served. One Sunday my daddy had enough of it and made the decision to never go back. My mom and I continued to go off and on, but not as often as before.

My parents were only seventeen and eighteen years old when I was born, so they themselves were still growing up as they took on the responsibility of parenthood. Daddy was making a living the best way he knew how—by providing for his family through working as a mechanic at the local garment factory and playing music on the weekends. You can't condemn a man for that. In my eyes, I had the coolest parents in town.

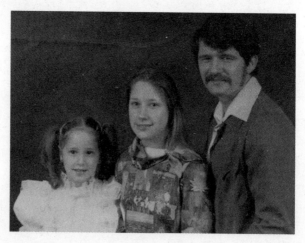

Me, Mom, and Dad

SEASON OF LIFE LESSON

I had a sweet childhood filled with lots of love. I was allowed to grow creatively, uniquely, and musically. I however didn't realize my soul was missing the fellowship and support of a church family until my husband and I joined Cornerstone Nashville Church a few years ago. I now get to experience the joy and the completeness it has brought to my life.

Whether we consciously know it or not, the foundation and strength we gain from being in relationship with other believers is a basic need for all creation. I believe this wholeheartedly.

You must prepare your ground before the storm, not in the middle of it. When the storm hits, you will need God's people to fight for you and gather around you in support.

I encourage everyone who hasn't already found himself or herself a Spirit-filled, Bible-teaching church family to do so. Serve with them, worship with them, grow with them, and do life with them. It will be one of the greatest blessings to your life's journey.

And I tell you, you are Peter, and on this rock I will build my church, and the gates of hell shall not prevail against it.

(Matthew 16:18 ESV)

When the storm has swept by, the wicked are gone, but the righteous stand firm forever. (Proverbs 10:25)

One of the many things my family taught me was how to work hard. I watched my dad work two jobs to take care of his family and build our first home. I watched my mom not only work outside the home but inside the home—taking care of the household and me.

They were both so young, but when I was born, they had to grow up really fast. I commend them both for teaching me so much and giving me more love than we had money.

Whatever you do, work at it with all your heart, as working for the Lord, not for human masters. (Colossians 3:23)

Find the song, *Louisiana Love Child*, on iTunes or Spotify under *Memarie Gayle*.

CHAPTER 2

Nashville

When I was twelve, Daddy decided it was time the family took a big step toward the family dream and move to the big city of Nashville. Coming from such a small town, it was a huge step for us indeed. I will never forget the day the three of us showed up at my aunt's house, which was full of all our friends and family yelling, "Surprise!"

It was a bittersweet day for us all. That's when it sank in for me that we were really moving to Nashville, far away from the only life I had ever known, and far away from everyone I had ever known or loved. I became really depressed just thinking about moving.

I have always been the overly-sensitive type, and it was no different in my childhood. I felt like my world was coming to an end, and I guess in reality it was—or at least the world that I had always known.

I grew up with only a cotton field between me and my Papaw Bud, Mamaw Inez, and Granny Ashley. So you see, they helped raise me. And for one year we even lived with my Granny Mary while we built our house. To say I was close to all my Grandparents is a huge understatement. My Grandparents were like second sets of parents to me. How could I leave all of them?

Let me tell you, it was not easy.

The first year in Nashville was scary for this small-town country girl. Besides dealing with the awkwardness of my age— which would have been plenty alone—I was entering junior high at a school where I knew no one, and I was the youngest in my class.

Yikes! I was coming from a school where I knew everyone, and I was entering that huge school filled with different cultures and new faces. It was a bit overwhelming to say the least. I was one frightened gal! I eventually settled in, but I never really felt at home.

Then during the summer before my eighth-grade year, my parents made another decision to move. My mom had received some attention from a record label based in North Carolina, and they needed us to move there. Yes, North Carolina! That seemed kind of weird considering we were living in Nashville— *Music City*.

I was not happy about that decision to move again. I lived in the small town of Baskin, Louisiana, for my entire twelve years of life, and now at thirteen I was moving again within a year's time. Well, as it turned out, in the whole scheme of life the move was actually a positive growing experience for me.

Rockford, North Carolina, was a smaller town than Nashville, so my school was a little smaller as well. That provided a little more familiar environment for me than the huge junior high school in Nashville. The new kids in Rockford were great, and I made friends very easily there. That made for a much happier eighth grade compared to my seventh-grade year.

Some of my new girlfriends even talked me into trying out for the following year's freshman cheer team. I was a little shy about it, but because my new friends were so encouraging and supportive, I ended up giving it a go and actually made the squad. I finally felt I was a part of something, and that was giving me back the confidence I had lost when we moved to Nashville.

I was excited about the next year and the new adventure with my new friends.

We rented a townhouse right next door to the businessman who put the whole record label together. He was an older, divorced man, so he lived alone in the townhouse connected to ours. It worked out well, because he and my dad could easily talk business and work until late if needed.

Things were going great! The record label landed my mom a fabulous country-music cruise, where she opened for Ricky Skaggs, The Whites, and Reba McEntire. My mom and dad knew they would be busy on the cruise, so they invited my Granny Mary to join us and keep me company.

I was so excited to be going on my first cruise, and I was getting to spend time with my Granny Mary! I had been missing her so much after the move to Nashville and North Carolina. We of course had a great time and made many wonderful memories!

Unfortunately, the excitement and comfort of our new little town was short lived. My dad always had a good sense for reading people, so once he started getting some vibes that were a bit off, he went into investigative mode. He went out and bought a little mini recorder and crawled up into the attic above the record label owner's townhouse and planted the recorder.

Yes, I know that was against the law! Yikes! My Mom and I laughed about it, and it was a miracle he didn't go to jail for that.

Well, low and behold, the guy was scamming us and all of the investors as well. He was scamming money from investors there in North Carolina and using most of it for other things instead of growing the record label. Shortly after the cruise, we ended up moving back to Nashville before my ninth-grade year even began. We packed up once again and headed back to Music City.

So there I was, the new girl once again, thrown into high school, starting over for a third time. I'm not sure how she did it, but my mom somehow talked me into trying out for the freshman cheerleading squad. I was so terrified, because I didn't know any of the girls, and I felt so alone. At least in North Carolina I had friends rooting me on and giving me support.

My mom felt that trying out for the cheerleading squad would be a great way for me to make friends, and if I could make the squad in North Carolina, then I could make the squad in Nashville. I somehow gathered all the courage a thirteen-year-old could gather and tried out for the team. Using all the new cheering skills that my sweet North Carolina girlfriends had taught me, I made the squad!

From that year on, I made the squad each year continuing through to my senior year of high school. My mom was right, it was a great way to make friends, and it actually helped my shyness just a bit. However, I never did quite shake the feeling of somehow being an outsider. I always felt like an outsider looking in at myself and on my social life.

As I made my way through figuring out high school, Mom and Dad made their way through figuring out the music business. My dad spent lots of time co-writing and making contacts in the *music biz*, while my mom worked full time. He kept lots of late hours as he continued to keep his eye on the dream.

Unfortunately, as my high school years went along, I could slowly see my parents drifting apart. And it was only a few months after I graduated from high school when my parents divorced.

The divorce was very hard on all of us. My mom ended up going back to Louisiana for several months to stay with Granny Mary while dealing with depression and anxiety, and my dad also was in deep depression. I felt more alone than I had ever felt in my life. My mom and dad were my safe place and my home. Even while moving from place to place, they were my constant.

We shared so much, including our love for music, and now all of that was gone.

While my family was falling apart, my boyfriend, who had been a long-time high school buddy, asked me to marry him at the wise age of eighteen years old. After my mom and dad divorced, I decided to marry him in hopes of conquering some of the loneliness I was feeling.

I had seen red flags of his jealousy while we were dating, but I ignored them. I was young and really had nothing to compare the experience to, so I followed through with the marriage. My dad was completely against it and refused to give me away at the wedding. And after that, our communication became nonexistent for the next two years.

Shortly after the wedding, the relationship I had with my husband became abusive—both mentally and physically. The physical abuse consisted of pushing, holding me down, screaming in my face, or throwing things. The bottom line was that we were both kids and had no idea what marriage was all about. He had his own personal demons that he was running from, and I had things I was running from too.

We were living in Murfreesboro and attending college. But I was not passionate about my major. I still had the dream of music in my heart. After two years of an unhealthy marriage, I finally gathered up enough courage to file for divorce and move back to Nashville to pursue my musical passions.

That was the first big decision I had ever made by that point in my life, and I gained a lot of strength from it. The courage and confidence it gave me really helped to move me forward into a new life of my own. I experienced an independence that I had never felt before, and I liked it!

Finally, for once in my life I was making decisions on my own and not letting the people around me make them for me—not my parents, and not a man in my life. At twenty-two years old, I owned my life, good or bad. That was when I truly finally felt like I had graduated into adulthood.

Shortly after my divorce, I started bartending at a local restaurant in Nashville, and I made new friends very quickly. After working there for a few months, I talked the owner into letting me host my own *Writer's Night* out on the patio. They paid me one hundred dollars every Friday night to host and to sing my own songs.

I invited other writers and had a great time doing what I loved, and I was actually getting paid for it. It also helped me to get past the fear of singing my own music in public. It was a great learning experience for sure. You could say I was cutting my musical teeth. That was officially my first paying gig.

Score!

Since that time in my life—fast forwarding to today—I have forgiven my ex, and I've moved forward. And he actually called me a few years ago to humbly apologize for any mistreatment and harm he caused me. I truly had forgiven him years ago, but he needed to voice his apology so he could also let go and move forward.

God calls us to forgive, and when we do, we ourselves are truly blessed. There is a peace that comes in our hearts that only forgiveness can deliver. One of the greatest things we can do for anyone in this life, including us, is to give the gift of forgiveness. It has more power to move us toward our godly purpose than almost anything I have encountered in this life.

Thank you, Jesus, for the power of forgiveness!

So back to 1995 . . .

After moving back to Nashville, I contacted my dad to let him know about the divorce. After that, we started to build our father-and-daughter relationship, and our common love for music was fostering a bond. I also began working part time for my dad's music company. We grew closer than we had ever been before.

Making music was something we always enjoyed together, so that was a special time in my life. He taught me all he knew about the business—copywriting, publishing, songwriting, recording, playing guitar, putting together a band, you name it. And I soaked it all up.

During that time, my dad was also busy writing and producing hits, so that was an exciting, busy time for him too. I remember going on a tour with him and Ken Mellons, an artist he was working with back then. That week on his tour bus was like a dream for me. I remember sleeping so well on the night drives—

just hearing the hum of the bus and dreaming of one day having my own tour bus and traveling from town to town, singing my heart out for sold-out crowds.

Soon I began dating a guy I met at the restaurant where I was bartending. He was finishing up his degree in college and working part time at the restaurant. I was twenty-two; and for the first time, I was living an independent life. I thought things were going great for my boyfriend and me until I found out he was cheating on me with another girl we worked with. I broke up with him immediately.

A couple of months later, though, he came running back to me begging for forgiveness and wanting to exclusively date me again. He would cook dinner for me, wine and dine me, declare over and over how sorry he was for what he had done, and tell me how much he loved me. He was really putting in the time to win me back. But I just could not seem to shake the trust issue.

I tried dating him again for a short time, but I ultimately decided it was not going to work out. However, just a few days after breaking off the relationship I started having some of the initial signs of being pregnant.

"Surely, I'm not pregnant! We were intimate only once during this short dating period. Surely this is not happening!" I told myself.

I took numerous pregnancy tests, and they all came back positive. I didn't know what to do. I was just starting to build back my relationship with my father, and I was finally working on my music. I knew that becoming a parent was going to mess it all up. I was devastated, and I was worried that my father would disown me again if he found out.

Some of my close girlfriends had gone through abortions, but I never expected to be in a position in which I would even consider such a thing. A close friend actually talked to me about it and offered to take me to a local clinic if I decided to do it. She had had an abortion just a few years earlier and knew how the process went.

At the time, I saw no other way but to terminate the pregnancy. I was consumed with fear of the unknown, fear of telling my father I was pregnant, and fear of raising a child at such a young age. And I did it.

I never blamed my father for the rash decision that I made then. He never even knew about it. I fully owned it, and needless to say, it became a decision that haunted me for many years to come. It was a life-changing, traumatic experience for me. You cannot realize the negative effects having an abortion will have on your life until later.

No one talked about abortion during those years. It wasn't a political topic, and there wasn't much information out there about it. I didn't even look at what I was doing as the taking of a life. In my mind it was way too early in the pregnancy for that.

Knowing what I do now, if a young girl were to ask my opinion on abortion today, I would tell her to absolutely not do it! There are so many other options—with adoption being at the top of my list.

SEASON OF LIFE LESSON

Young adulthood was a hard season of growth. I gained my wings of independence but learned how independence can also lead us to a dark place if it isn't grounded by the Word of God. I learned how to stand on my own two feet and make decisions for myself, some of which affected the rest of my life—some positively and some negatively.

I was a scared young girl who made a horrifically bad decision out of fear. I was tormented for many years with guilt and shame, but today I live free from it. I ran from God for a few years hiding my face of shame from Him, but God is patient, and He is relentless in His pursuit of us. The grace shown to me by my Savior, Jesus Christ, taught me to finally give grace to myself, and the chains of that sin were broken.

I forever live in gratitude that His blood covers my sin.

If we confess our sins, he is faithful and just to forgive us our sins and to cleanse us from all unrighteousness.   (1 John 1:9 ESV)

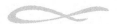

You can find the song, *God Be with Me*, on iTunes or Spotify under *Memarie Gayle*.

CHAPTER 3

Lessons in Fear

For a couple of years, I continued to work part time for my dad. I strived hard to prove to him that I was really serious about a music career. He finally agreed to produce an album for me, and I was so excited!

Dad's career was in full swing, so in order for him to agree to produce an album for me, he had to make sure I was ready to work hard. I was ready, and I was excited to get started on the journey together!

After finding a job with a great salary and benefits in the marketing department of a local software company, I decided to quit my bartending job. It allowed me to work on my music at night and on the weekends. And there, I met a man, whom I began dating, and we soon became engaged. He had many great qualities that anyone would look for in a mate—great job, great family, nice guy, and good looks.

We were eventually engaged to be married, but I could never seem to commit to setting a wedding date. There was something missing in that relationship, even though I could not quite put my finger on what it was. I just knew he wasn't the man I was supposed to marry. But simply out of fear of being alone, I think I held on to that relationship longer than I should have.

I clearly needed courage to make the right decisions, and I gained that courage in a rather unique way. It was when I got my scuba-diving certificate and went on my first scuba trip. For the scuba trip, we set to sea on a fifty-foot sailboat for five days—with scuba diving day and night. The night dive was the scariest and most magical thing I had ever experienced in my life. I will never forget it!

The ocean was pitch black, and there were three large sea turtles swimming around the boat. All the other divers had jumped in for their dive, but I was still standing on the edge of the boat gathering my courage to jump. I felt the fear all through my body. Frozen with fear, I wasn't about to jump into that water for anything or anybody.

I'm not sure how it happened, but after what seemed like an eternity, I pushed the fear away and made the plunge into the black ocean!

As I descended down into the waters, the ocean opened up into a magical, colorful underwater world. Pictures and videos I had seen did not do the beautiful, submerged landscape justice. Swimming in the warm Caribbean Ocean was amazing, and seeing all the wonderful things God created in that underwater wonderland was breathtaking.

I was elated with joy when I returned to the boat after the dive. I had overcome a fear, and I had witnessed so much beauty from conquering that fear. As crazy as it was, that feeling of overcoming fear was what gave me the courage to end my engagement. If I could defeat the fear of the ocean, surely I could overcome the fear of being alone and breaking off a relationship that just wasn't right for me. So that's what I did.

SEASON OF LIFE LESSON

Wow, I am so glad I conquered the fear of that ocean! Overcoming my fear that night taught me a valuable lesson in how fear can hold us back, and how conquering fear can propel us forward. But that was just one of many lessons I learned in fighting fear—with more yet to come. And you'll understand that more fully as you continue reading.

Thank you, God, for teaching me that life lesson in such a unique and unexpected way.

Have I not commanded you? Be strong and courageous. Do not be afraid; do not be discouraged, for the Lord your God will be with you wherever you go. (Joshua 1:9)

Therefore do not worry about tomorrow, for tomorrow will worry about itself. Each day has enough trouble of its own. (Matthew 6:34)

CHAPTER 4

Thankful in the Storm

Neill is a man who worked for the same company I did, but in a different department. He was a really good guy, and we became friends while working there.

A few months after I went to work there, a group of us at work decided to go hear a blues band in downtown Nashville. At the last-minute, Neill called to let me know everyone else had bowed out, but he was still up for going if I was. To make a long story short, that night indirectly ended up being our first date.

We had the best time together. We laughed, laughed, and laughed even more. That was our first time hanging out away from work, and I hadn't realized it until that night just how similar our personalities were. From that night forward we started dating and were inseparable. I really feel like God brought him to me. He had a great heart!

We laughed a lot together, we could talk about anything with one another, and he brought calm to my creative craziness. There was something different about our relationship than any other I had experienced. There was a peace in knowing that I was where I was supposed to be. We fell in love quickly and were married a year later.

About two years into our marriage, my music career really started to take off. I was writing songs and playing music constantly. I was giving it my all, because I felt it was *now or never*. My dad started his own record label with investment dollars intact, and musically speaking I was *readier* than ever. We released my first single, and I quit my marketing job to begin touring immediately.

It was an exciting time and a busy few years for me.

I was doing radio and media tours all over the country, walking red carpets, shooting music videos, doing photo shoots, and opening for A-list acts. The first song we had success with was a Christian country song that my dad wrote, called *What If He's Right*.

He literally was awakened by the Holy Spirit one night while in Memphis and wrote the entire song in the middle of the night. The single went to *number one* on the Christian country charts, and it was the longest running number one song in that genre at the time.

I went on to have several other songs hit the Top 40 on the Billboard country charts. In the midst of all the excitement, I was very focused on what was next instead of enjoying what was happening in the moment. Looking back on it all now, I realize just how blessed I was. I am so thankful for the opportunities I had and the memories I treasure.

The success my dad and I had together is something I will cherish forever.

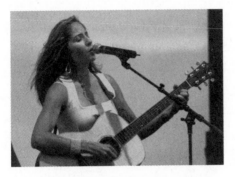

Me opening for Tracy Lawrence

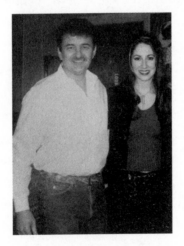

Me and my dad

During that time of my success in the music business, I was on the road almost as much or more than I was at home. It seemed I was on the verge of breaking into stardom, but all the while, my marriage was suffering for it. Neill and I grew farther and farther apart as I traveled more and more. I could feel my marriage slipping away in 2008, and I felt my dreams slipping away as well.

I was in my thirties, and although I had some success, I had not reached my ultimate goals in the music business. My dad also lost his investor for the label and had to downsize the company. I was scared—to say the least.

Neill had talked to me about shopping for a new label for quite some time, and I was starting to think that it might just be the time to do that. With my dad losing funding and my career at a point where I felt I had to keep the momentum going, I decided to leave my dad's record label.

My dad took that decision really personally—to the heart. He felt I was not being loyal to him. And what I hoped to be a peaceful parting of ways and a positive move for my career turned into a really ugly parting.

After my dad had time to stew on the idea of me leaving the record label, I received a surprising letter from him. He expressed his feelings on the matter of me leaving, and he didn't *hold back*. I never wanted my dad to take my leaving personal. For me it was a business decision. And whether right or wrong for my career, it was my decision.

I completely shut down after that day. I closed myself off from him and everyone else. It was like the window to my soul closed shut. Nothing could get in or out. My dad and I didn't speak for a couple of years. He didn't reach out to me, and I didn't reach out to him.

That lack of communication with my dad put me in a very unhealthy emotional state. I began to hold on to bitterness, and I closed myself off from any love that was in my life—including the love of my husband. In a twisted way, I think I blamed Neill for the downfall and the assumption that I had lost my dad's love once again.

At the time, I felt that if I had stayed on his record label, my dad would still love me, and we would still be in communication. I felt that if I had not let Neill's opinion sway me, I could also possibly be in a better position with my career. I had all those thoughts running around in my head, and I became angry at the world.

When I look back at the person I became during that time, it is as though I am looking through a keyhole at an entirely different person. Bitterness will change you, my friend. I was living proof of that. I became a shell of myself—void of emotion—and I decided that no one was going to hurt me like my dad had hurt me. So I pushed everyone away.

I ended up stepping outside my marriage during that time, which further added to my anger and isolation. Then I was not only angry with my dad but also with myself. I was the girl who never even cheated on a boyfriend in high school or college. I wondered how I let myself get to that vulnerable state. The once confident girl turned into a woman filled with shame, hurt, anger, and guilt.

I was the girl all her friends turned to when they needed advice for a problem. But then I not only wanted to run away from my life, I wanted to run away from myself. I asked myself how I could do that to Neill. So much confusion cluttered my mind and spirit.

My mind became the devil's playground. I felt that nothing or no one could save me from the self-destructive state I was in—not even God. Even today the thoughts can come to me: "How could

He save me when I was running from Him too? How could He forgive me when I couldn't even forgive myself?" Yet He did!

I had my first-ever anxiety/panic attack the night I told Neill of my infidelity. My body began to shake, and I felt like I could not breath as I sobbed uncontrollably. I felt shame and guilt rush into me like never before. I was so overwhelmed with guilt that I could not see through it. It was like the guilt had a grip on me, and it was not letting go anytime soon.

As the weeks passed, my guilt only grew stronger, and the only way out that I could see was to run. I walked around in a haze for months. It was like I was in a room filled with thick smoke, and that room was my life. I had lost my dad, and now I was losing my husband.

Divorce proceedings started, and I moved into a tiny apartment and tried to put the pieces of my life back together. I was broken and looking to the world for comfort. I guess I felt that getting away on my own would clear my thoughts and help me to move forward in my life, but everything I did only caused me to feel more alone and more depressed.

The shame and guilt caused me to push God farther and farther away from me. I didn't feel like God even wanted to be near me. That was the lie Satan used to keep me from the love and comfort of my heavenly Father. I continued to have horrific anxiety attacks over the next few months, and I even began having thoughts of suicide.

Many times, God uses His people to reach down into our darkness and speak to us. My grandmother was one of those people God used to speak to me during that season of my life. She told me, "When you are feeling overwhelmed, start thanking

God in that moment for anything at all that you are thankful for. It could even be the smallest, simplest things."

I will never forget what she said. "Take for instance your eyelashes. God created them so the sun would not hurt your eyes, dust can't get in them as easily, and the raindrops can't fall onto your eyeballs."

We had a good laugh over that, but it was also the best advice anyone could give me at that moment in time. Sometimes we go through things—times when we feel there is *NOTHING* to celebrate—but there is always something to be thankful for.

I was definitely thankful for my Granny Mary. She was definitely something in my life worth celebrating.

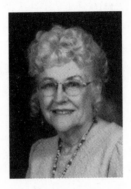

Granny Mary

This may sound silly, but I had a precious Pomeranian named Goldie, and she always woke me up in the morning. She slept with me in my bed, and she woke me up licking my face and wagging her tail to go outside. I decided that she was something for me to be thankful for every single day. She brought a smile to my face first thing every morning. Every morning while walking her, I thanked God for all the things I was thankful for.

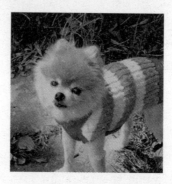

Goldie–my little angel

Even though most days I still felt hopeless, I followed my Granny Mary's advice. I could still think of the smallest of blessings and thank God for them. And that began to soften my heart and put me on a road toward healing. It was the first time in my life I consciously began each day with a thankful heart.

Thank you, Granny Mary, for teaching me how to have a thankful heart even through some of the hardest seasons of life!

SEASON OF LIFE LESSON

God gives us warning signs when we are heading in a direction that is outside of His will for us. He throws up red flags and caution signs, but I looked past them and kept heading in the opposite direction. I thought I could handle being in tempting situations, because I wasn't a cheater.

It's true what they say: "When you walk too close to the fire you are bound to get burned." Sometimes the sin we think we are the most unlikely to commit can be just the one Satan uses to snare us.

It is so important to establish boundaries in order to protect your marriage. Just like other relationships in life, the marriage relationship is in constant motion—with partners either growing together or growing apart. If you are not making a conscious effort to make deposits into your marriage, it will surely grow apart.

In times of disappointment and struggle, you are vulnerable to temptation. When boundaries are set on the front end, it closes the gap for many of those temptations during vulnerable times.

Therefore what God has joined together, let no one separate.

(Mark 10:9)

Secular psychologists say that gratitude is an antidote to negative emotions like envy, jealousy, anger, greed, hostility, and impatience. Of course, God already knew that. Thankfulness slowly brought me out of depression. Being thankful even in the middle of what felt like a desert was the greatest lesson I learned. I would venture to say it is one of the greatest lessons I will ever learn in this life!

Give thanks in all circumstances; for this is God's will for you in Christ Jesus.   (1 Thessalonians 5:18)

That season was so heavy with fear that I decided I really wanted to try to rid my life of it and consciously choose to live in faith. My new year's resolution/motto that year became "Choose faith over fear in the new year."

I remember texting that to all my friends and family, and I have carried this motto throughout my life ever since.

So do not fear, for I am with you; do not be dismayed, for I am your God. I will strengthen you and help you; I will uphold you with my righteous right hand. (Isaiah 41:10)

I sought the Lord, and he answered me and delivered me from all my fears. (Psalm 34:4 ESV)

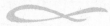

You can find my song, *I Don't Want to Hurt You Anymore*, on iTunes or Spotify under *Memarie Gayle*.

You can find my song, *What If He's Right*, on *https://fearlessmemories.com/*. This was a number one song written by my dad.

CHAPTER 5

Made to Create

While I was living in a tiny apartment and going through that horrific time in my life, God kept showing me a picture in my mind. I would dream of it at night and think of it during the day. I knew it was from God, but I really didn't have a clue what it meant.

The dream was of a dark, barren field of snow. No one was around, and it was a quiet, peaceful place. In the distance I could see a tree with lots of dead, white limbs. As I walked closer to the tree in the snow, I could see one ripe cherry hanging from the tree limb. It was brilliant, shiny red!

That image would not get out of my head, so I went to Hobby Lobby and bought a large canvas and some paint. I slowly painted the picture over the next few days. I'm not a painter by the way, but I had to get it out of my head. As I painted, God revealed His message to me.

As His revelation became clearer to me, I could feel the comfort of the Holy Spirit wrapping around me. The dark field of snow was my life. The dead tree was the state I was currently in. And the ripe cherry was me—truly me! It was *the me* God saw—the one He created me to be.

This became my hope.

The next two years became a bit of push-and-pull. I would move two steps forward, then two steps back. I was growing in my faith but still holding on to my own will. I didn't know it then, but forgiveness was the key I needed to unlock my heart. I couldn't forgive myself for my actions that led to my divorce, and I couldn't forgive my dad for our strained relationship.

I'd had an idea for a song for months, but I would not allow myself to write it. It was about my divorce, and I didn't want to hash over all that pain again, so I pushed it away like everything else. But for whatever reason, one particular night I decided to finally get out my guitar and write the song, *Ghost*.

I worked on it for several nights through a lot of tears and a lot of soul-searching. It was tough going, but I finished it. When I did finally finish it, I felt this great sense of relief and accomplishment. I allowed myself to feel the pain of the divorce and let the tears fall. There was something about writing the song that helped clear out some of the smoke in the room of my life.

Throughout the writing it was just God and me, creating and healing. Because some time had passed since the divorce, with God's help I was able to look at it from another perspective and get on the other side of the pain. And I was able to purge my way through the emotions.

Through the process of writing the song, I allowed the creativity to heal me. For me, the song, *Ghost*, represents a turning point in my life. I decided right then and there that it was time to move on and stop holding on to my past. That marked the beginning of my forgiveness.

God really continued working on me over the next few months. I could feel Him working in my life, but I was still not ready to completely give over my life to Him. I always considered myself a Christian, but I never really understood what it was to live my life for God and have a real, personal relationship with Him.

Christmas was usually spent with family in Louisiana, and that year was no different. I stayed with my Granny Mary, and I was also going to visit my Mamaw Inez (Daddy's mom). My dad and I were still not on speaking terms, so I called Mamaw Inez to let her know I was coming over.

I knew Dad would be there visiting for Christmas, and I wasn't sure if he would want to see me or not. When I pulled into her driveway my dad walked out alone and walked right up to my Jeep. He asked if we could take a walk. We walked down the old gravel road that held so many memories for both of us—where both of us had grown up.

My Mamaw Inez still lived in the house he grew up in, and across the field was the house that he built and we lived in for most of my childhood. So there we were, walking together, but at a time in our life when we had gone over a year without even speaking.

We reminisced of good memories as we walked. Then he told me that no matter what he felt or thought about my decisions, he still loved me. And I told him the same.

He told me he never stopped loving me. I needed to hear that, but I was also waiting for an apology that I felt I deserved. I didn't get it, so while I left there feeling somewhat better, I still held on to what I thought I needed from him.

A few months later, while I was sitting on the same couch where I wrote the song, *Ghost*, God began to work in me again. I realized that my dad was my dad, and I could no longer expect him to be something other than who he was. I either had to accept him as he was or continue to keep him at a distance.

The bitterness toward my dad that I had held on to slowly began to disappear in that instant, and all I felt was love. I began to cry and miss him and forget all the things that held me back from reaching out to him over the last two years. I just wanted a relationship with my daddy, and it didn't matter how little or how much. I just wanted my daddy in my life.

That night I decided I was ready to forgive him. I sent an e-mail message to him before going to bed and asked him if he would like to have lunch that week. To my surprise, he promptly sent a message back to me the next day and said that he would love to have lunch.

We went to lunch that week, and we both agreed to be open and honest with each other in order to get everything out on the table. After we talked that day, we decided to leave everything in the past and move forward.

I'm so thankful that God softened and opened my heart to my dad that night. It allowed me to reach out to him and begin mending our relationship. For the next three years my dad and I continued to build back our relationship as we became closer and closer.

SEASON OF LIFE LESSON

Creativity is healing. I learned this through the painting I did of the dead cherry tree in the snow and through writing the song, *Ghost*. The painting was not a masterpiece by any means, but the process of producing it was the greatest gift to me.

I've always had a talent for music and writing songs. And I've always known that music was therapeutic for me, but what I didn't know is how God could work through it. What I want everyone to understand is that you do not need to be talented in the arts to gain healing, therapeutic gifts from it. Just create. You don't even have to show anyone. Just do it!

I believe God works through creativity. After all, He is the ultimate Creator—the Creator of the Universe.

In the beginning God created the heaven and the earth.
(Genesis 1:1 KJV)

The hope God showed me through my painting also helped me forgive myself for the downfall of my marriage. God still saw me as that shiny red fruit hanging on the dead, barren tree. Where I was seeing darkness in my life, God saw the light still there inside me.

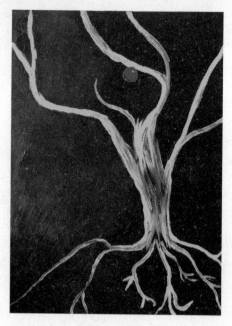

My painting

Sometimes in life we have to stop expecting people to be who we want them to be. We have to either accept people for who they are or move on. If I had continued to be stubborn and hold out for my dad to give me what I thought I needed from him emotionally, we might have never rebuilt our relationship.

Sometimes we must set aside our pride and decide what is more important in our lives. For me, the relationship with my dad was much more important. God can soften hearts and break down walls if we allow Him to work in us.

Forgiveness was the key to unlock my heart in that season. The painting showed me how God saw me, which allowed me to forgive myself. Then once I forgave myself, forgiving my dad was much easier. Bitterness and an unforgiving heart will cause your well of love to dry up. By holding on to unforgiveness, you put a lid on your well of love.

Just remove the lid, and forgiveness and love will flow out of you like pure water.

> *Get rid of all bitterness, rage and anger, brawling and slander, along with every form of malice. Be kind and compassionate to one another, forgiving each other, just as in Christ God forgave you.* (Ephesians 4:31-32)

You can find the song, *Ghost*, on iTunes or Spotify under *Memarie Gayle*.

CHAPTER 6

Faith over Fear

Just a few weeks before that lunch with Dad, I met a man who was also a singer/songwriter. We hit it off right away and soon began dating. Over the following six months, our relationship grew more serious. I felt like that was my chance to get things right. Where I had failed with Neill, I wanted to do things right with my new boyfriend.

We began playing music together and traveling across the country. He was very anxious for us to start our life together. We became engaged to marry, and he wanted me to move with him back to his home state of Michigan. There were lots of musical opportunities there in the northern part of the state—like playing yacht clubs, country clubs, and resorts.

I was kind of over the Nashville music scene, and it seemed like a great opportunity to have a fresh start, both personally and musically.

Things progressed quickly, and before long we were moving to northern Michigan. And we were engaged shortly thereafter. For the first few months in northern Michigan everything seemed great. We were making a name for ourselves throughout the area and playing as many shows as we could fit into our calendar.

In addition to music, I started a handmade jewelry business. I had always designed and made jewelry for my stage shows, and as more people started asking about how they could purchase my jewelry, I began to sell pieces here and there.

One night at one of our shows I met a lovely couple who owned a home decor/gift boutique in the small lake town where we lived. The lady inquired about a necklace I was wearing, and that ended up being the first boutique to carry *Fearless Memories Jewelry*. From there, I placed my designs in three more stores in the area.

On the opposite end of the spectrum was our personal life. As the months went on, I started seeing red flags in my fiancé's personality. It began with verbal and emotional abuse and escalated to him throwing objects (whatever he could grab) that seemed to always land in my direction—many times leaving bruises. He always said it was accidental, but after it happened many times, I knew it was no accident.

He also began using my past mistakes against me and tried his best to make me feel like I was inferior to him in every way. Nothing was ever good enough. No matter how hard I tried, I could not make him happy.

Abusers themselves have such a low self-esteem that they need to beat someone else's down in order to build up their own esteem. That's such a twisted way of thinking! I had never known someone who was such an extreme narcissist. He was so extreme that I had to *Google it,* and yes, there was his picture right beside the word *narcissist.* Ha!

One night in the midst of an argument he threw me against the wall with his hands tightly around my neck. He squeezed tighter and tighter while yelling in my face that he was going to kill me. I had never seen so much evil in one person's eyes. Once he let go I grabbed a knife from the kitchen counter and yelled for him to leave me alone.

Evidently the look in my eye told him that I would protect myself with whatever means needed, because he quickly ran outside into the mudroom. I did finally put the knife back in the butcher block and sat down to gather myself. Once he came back inside, the argument continued.

He then threw me on the floor and began to hit and kick me. All I knew to do was lay curled up in the corner and try to shield the blows. You would think a woman would leave after that kind of abuse. And that is what I thought too—until I was that woman. The opposite is actually the reality in most cases.

I was more afraid than ever to leave, because I knew what he was capable of, and I was terrified of what more he might do. So I stayed, and I prayed.

Shortly after that incident I found out my dad was fighting a rare blood cancer. He had been having many unexplainable symptoms for a few years with no diagnosis until then. I will never forget. I was enjoying the sun on the deck of our Cobalt boat on Lake Michigan the day I received the phone call with the news.

It was a rare, pleasant day, because my fiancé was in a relaxed mood, and I was enjoying the peace and quiet of soaking up the sun. The mood quickly changed after that call, though. I was in shock, because my dad was always the strong one, the one who was never sick, and he always seemed younger than his age.

The news of his illness, along with lots of prayer, actually gave me the push and the strength I needed to leave my abusive relationship. We had several larger show contracts to fulfill over the next couple of months, so I decided to stay just long enough to meet those obligations while I devised my plan to leave.

I told my boyfriend I was anxious to get back to Nashville to make sure my dad was okay. As far as he was concerned, we were just taking a little break from our relationship, and I would be back with him as soon as I could.

I could never tell him I had decided to leave him for good. After all, just a few nights before I left, he had locked me outside the house in knee-deep snow for a couple of hours after trying to talk me out of leaving one last time. When I told him I had not changed my mind, he literally pushed me out the door and locked it. That was one of the scariest nights leading up to the day I left.

The most dangerous time for a woman who is escaping an abusive relationship is during the leaving process. I prayed for God's protection every day during that time.

On the morning I had planned to leave, we woke up to a nasty snowstorm. Of course my boyfriend used the weather to try to keep me there a few more days, but I had made up my mind that nothing would stop me from leaving, not even a blizzard. I continued to tell him that I would be back, but I had to get to Nashville to be with my dad.

To my surprise, he was on his best behavior on the day I left, and he even shed a few regretful tears for some of the things he had done. He told me he loved me and said he wanted me to come back to him soon. I said goodbye and drove down the long snow-filled driveway.

As my wheels hit the road, I could feel the weight lifting. It was as if the snow floating in the air was carrying my tears to heaven. I knew in that moment I was going to be okay. As the tears flowed, I thanked God for the next few miles. Those were tears of relief, tears of joy, and tears of praise.

I will sing God's praise forever, for He takes what Satan means for evil and turns it into good.[2]

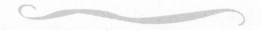

SEASON OF LIFE LESSON

The biggest lesson of that season was learning how to trust God completely. When I moved to northern Michigan, I was taken away from all of my family and friends to a remote place where the only person I knew was my fiancé.

When the abuse started, I had to gain my strength from Christ. My self-esteem had been beaten down so much that the anxiety attacks came flooding back. After we had a fight all I knew to do was read the Word, pray, and talk to God. Slowly through growing my personal relationship with Christ, He whispered into my spirit, and the lies that the enemy was telling me slowly went away.

My abuser wanted me to feel like I was nothing without him, but God helped me to believe I was everything through Christ.

---

2 "You intended to harm me, but God intended it for good to accomplish what is now being done, the saving of many lives" (Genesis 50:20).

Where my own strength ran short, God's strength filled me up again, and I was made strong. Through reading God's Word, the Lord spoke to me in an almost audible voice, telling me, "You deserve more than this!"

That soaked into my spirit, and it is what gave me courage like I had never felt before. The strength of God is what sustained me in the days leading up to leaving the abusive relationship, and it sustained me as I drove out of Michigan through the terrible snowstorm.

A message taught by Christian leader, Dr. Sam Chand, comes to my mind. He said:

1. Get up—no excuses or blame.
2. Pick up—pick up and own it and be done with it—carry your own cross.
3. Walk up—walk away from people and things and habits that hold you back from God's purpose in your life.
4. Keep up—once you've made the change and you are following Jesus, you continue that path and feed your faith to keep you rooted, so you can keep up.

I wrote a song just a year prior to leaving that relationship called Faith Over Fear. During that season of my life the words in the song came to life for me as I used my faith to conquer my fear in getting out of my abusive relationship. Once again God spoke to me through my creativity and helped me to heal.

He gives strength to the weary, and to him who lacks might he increases power. (Isaiah 40:29 NASB)

Do not fear, for I am with you; do not anxiously look about you, for I am your God. I will strengthen you, surely I will help you, surely I will uphold you with My righteous right hand.

(Isaiah 41:10 NASB)

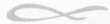

You can find the songs, *Faith Over Fear* and *Broken Beautiful*, on iTunes or Spotify under *Memarie Gayle*.

CHAPTER 7

The Prophecy

When I arrived in Nashville my mom and stepfather had decorated their home with a welcome-home banner and balloons. That made my homecoming a special day to remember. It took me at least a month to decompress, but as the weight of the abusive relationship lifted, I began to finally feel like myself again.

The *self* I had lost during that two-year relationship was slowly returning, but it was a better version of the one I had before. This self was the one God created me to be—confident, free from shame and guilt, and armed with a new passion for Christ. My relationship with my Creator was the closest it had ever been in my life. I felt His hand on me, and I was learning more and more every day about how to let the Holy Spirit lead and guide my steps.

After moving back to Nashville, I made the decision to really work on my jewelry brand and to grow my business. That included many, many trips to Hobby Lobby before I gained my business license and started wholesale ordering. One particular day while at Hobby Lobby shopping for jewelry supplies, a lady came up from behind me and tapped me on the shoulder.

"Excuse me," she said, "Are you in the ministry?"

I asked her to repeat what she said, because I wasn't sure if I understood her correctly.

"Are you in the ministry?" she repeated.

"No, I'm not," I replied.

"Are you sure?" she said.

"No, I'm not," I repeated.

"Well you have God shining all over you. I just knew you were in the ministry." She went on to tell me that God prompted her to come over to me and tell me that year was going to be a great year of blessings for me.

Chills ran all over me, and I knew in that moment that the Holy Spirit was there among us. I thanked her, and then I had to go out to my car to have a good, happy cry and thank Jesus for the wonderful word from that lady I had never seen before.

My jewelry business really started taking off a few weeks later, and I was able to land a few boutique wholesale accounts. Once my business started picking up, I decided I wanted to do a ministry to help abused women. So I started the *Faith Over Fear Ministry* and held my first workshop at a domestic abuse shelter in Franklin, Tennessee.

In my workshop I helped the women make *Faith Over Fear* bracelets as I told them my story of abuse. I ministered to them with music that proclaims how God saw me through and helped me get out of an abusive relationship. It was just as much of a blessing to me as it was for the women there.

Telling my story for the first time was a large part of my healing and moving forward. A few days after the workshop, I was sitting at my mom's kitchen counter working on my *Fearless Memories* website. The Holy Spirit brought something back to my mind that the lady in the Hobby Lobby store had said to me.

She asked me if I was in the ministry. I had not even thought about one particular aspect of what she said until right then sitting in my mom's home. In that moment, God was telling me I was on track and in His will. I joyfully thanked God for giving me that confirmation.

Shortly after arriving back in Nashville, my mom told me she had been in contact with my ex-husband, Neill, through e-mail a few months earlier. She had purchased for him a really nice leather Bible years ago, while we were married, and never had a chance to give it to him after the divorce. She decided to send an e-mail message to him and get his address so she could mail the Bible to him.

She had sent the message almost a year prior to his response. He apologized to her for taking so long to get back to her. He gave her his address and proceeded to ask how I was doing. She told him I had moved to Michigan and was engaged. He said he had a disturbing dream about me the previous night, and he just needed to know I was okay.

Once I heard about Neill's dream, I had a strong urge to call him. It had been over two years since we had seen or spoken to one another, so I was a little nervous about it. But with my new-found strength, I pushed through the fear and gave him a call.

We talked for over two hours. I was anxious to ask him about the dream he had, so I got right to the point and asked him.

He told me the dream started with him walking into a house where he found me lying on the floor crying and terribly beaten. After he saw me on the floor, a man suddenly walked in the door very upset! He confronted Neill, and they got into an altercation. Then the dream abruptly ended.

He told me he woke up with a lingering fear for my safety and needed to know I was okay. That is when he finally responded to my mom's message about the Bible and asked her how I was doing. I could not believe my ears!

I really felt God had given him that dream to connect us back together. I asked Neill if he would be willing to see me. I also asked if he would be willing to have an open mind to see if there was a possibility of a second chance if everything went well.

I had no idea I was going to ask him that during our first conversation. I was just calling to ask about the dream. But the next thing I knew, I was asking about much more than that. I felt God had brought me back to Nashville to save me—and also to give me the life I was meant to have.

I was letting God lead me, and I was leaving fear behind. Neill said he was willing to give it a try, and we decided to meet for dinner and catch up—with no expectations. We also decided it was best to wait at least a few weeks to allow me time to tie up some loose ends and have a little more time to heal from the toxic emotions of the abusive relationship.

Three weeks later, we had talked on the phone a handful of times, and we were ready to meet up. The night we went to dinner, the manager of the restaurant came over to our table and said to us, "You guys win the award for the most romantic table here tonight." We looked up at him and both just smiled.

I was a bit surprised because we had not kissed or even held hands that night! We were just engaged in our conversation.

Evidently, he saw something in our eyes as we caught up on each other's lives. After that dinner we talked every day on the phone and saw each other every weekend for a year. We reconnected during that time and also got to know the new people we had grown into. I prayed that God would heal our hearts and continue to nurture our relationship.

As we grew closer, the desire inside me to make it right with Neill's family also grew. One day while visiting Neill's dad and his wife, they both told me they had forgiven me and were very happy Neill and I were dating. That was music to my heart—and such a relief to know they were supporting us.

After that, I still felt God was tugging at my heart to talk to Neill's mom and his sister. I made a promise to God that I would do that, but I wasn't sure when or how it would happen. I had been around them only a couple of times. They were both respectful to me each time, but I could feel a tension there.

I completely understood that tension, took responsibility for it, and wanted to do my part to break its chains. I knew that if God had brought me that far He would see it through to completion.

One Sunday night after having dinner with Neill's family, his mom, his sister, and I were in the kitchen cleaning up. I felt the voice of God whisper it was time. I acted quickly before I had time to talk myself out of it and before fear had time to creep in on me. I humbled myself and told them both that I would not blame them for hating me. After all, I hated myself for a long time until God intervened and allowed me to forgive myself.

They then told me they did not hate me, and it was evident to me that God had been working His miracles within their hearts as well. With every tear shed, the walls crumbled down. Praise Jesus for the power of His love and the power of forgiveness!

My relationship with Neill's family continues to grow, and it is great today. I am so thankful for their forgiving hearts, and I'm so thankful to have been welcomed back into their wonderful family.

It wasn't too long after that day when Neill asked me to marry him. And we remarried on June 22, 2014 on the beach at Laguna Beach, California. We had a simple, private ceremony that included Neill, me, the minister, and a photographer to document the day. It was perfect! The only other day in my life that I felt that much joy was our first wedding day.

SEASON OF LIFE LESSON

Many times throughout that year, the words of the lady I met in Hobby Lobby rang in my ear. I'm not sure if she was an angel or if she was simply a messenger God put in my life that day. Either way, I knew God was in it, and He got His message across loud and clear.

I remarried Neill. I regained the family I had lost. I was able to grow my jewelry business beyond what I had in Michigan. And, yes indeed, I was called to ministry through my jewelry business and my music.

Through God all things are possible.[3] The prophetic words of the lady in Hobby Lobby strengthened my faith with the

---

3 "Jesus looked at them and said, "With man this is impossible, but not with God; all things are possible with God" (Mark 10:27).

supernatural ways of our living God. He is still working through people today just as He did in the days when the Bible was written. He is the same yesterday, today, and forever.[4] Amen.

> *We also have the prophetic message as something completely reliable, and you will do well to pay attention to it, as to a light shining in a dark place, until the day dawns and the morning star rises in your hearts.* (2 Peter 1:19)

Not long after Neill and I remarried, his mom told me that after we divorced she had prayed God would bring Neill a good, godly woman. I had also been praying the same for Neill. She followed up by saying I was the answer to her prayer. What she said meant more to me than she will ever know.

God answered our prayers in a way we could have never imagined. Thank you, Jesus, for molding me into that godly woman we had both prayed for.

> *Therefore I tell you, whatever you ask for in prayer, believe that you have received it, and it will be yours.* (Mark 11:24)

> *So the Lord blessed Job in the second half of his life even more than the beginning.* (Job 42:12a NLT)

God revealed in our experiences that He not only still speaks today through people, He also still gives people dreams. If God had not given Neill the vision in his dream, I'm not sure I would have ever had the courage to call him. I believe that was just one more piece of God's plan to put our marriage back together. God works ALL things according to His purpose.

---

4 "Jesus Christ is the same yesterday and today and forever" (Hebrews 13:8).

"In the last days," God says, "I will pour out my Spirit on all people. Your sons and daughters will prophesy, your young men will see visions, your old men will dream dreams."   (Acts 2:17)

You can find my song, *I Live for the One*, on iTunes or Spotify under *Memarie Gayle*.

CHAPTER 8

Daddy

My dad was still battling cancer, and Dad had a bone marrow transplant right after Neill and I remarried. His sister Glenda tested positive as a donor, and she was more than willing to donate bone marrow for the transplant. Dad's attitude was very positive, and he felt that he was going to beat cancer.

Dad was doing well after the transplant, except for the weakness from the chemotherapy. But once the bone marrow transplant started taking effect and his stem cells slowly started producing healthy cells, he became weaker and weaker. It seemed that if there was a side effect or a setback to be had, he had it.

He developed *Graft-Versus-Host* disease, which meant some of his body was rejecting the bone marrow. At the time, the doctors started giving him medication to help with the problem. And before long, it all balanced out, and he was back on track to recovery. But his recovery was short lived, because he again developed Graft-Versus-Host, which called for an emergency surgery to remove a section of his colon.

After the surgery he was forced to wear a colostomy bag, which was very upsetting to him. One thing I remember him always saying was that he never wanted to wear a colostomy bag, so that was a major setback for him—not only physically but also mentally.

The recovery time following surgery was longer than hoped, and his muscles further weakened. He was still on numerous medications for the bone marrow transplant, and now he was healing from major surgery. During that time his muscles atrophied to the point he was no longer strong enough to walk.

He began physical therapy, but the progress was very slow and ineffective. After multiple setbacks, he was dealing with serious depression.

It was also getting more difficult for his wife to take care of him at home by herself, and a sweet older couple at the church they attended offered for them to come live with them while he recovered. They had wheelchair access at their home because they had previously taken care of a family member who needed that kind of arrangement.

I remember the first day we moved my dad into their house. I stayed there with Dad all day. He broke down like I had never seen before. He was always so strong, but the disease and complications from it had broken him. I think having to move out of his own home and have someone else help really took a hit to his pride.

We just hugged and both cried. I left there feeling helpless and not knowing of anything I could do for him except pray.

I visited him several times a week while he was there. After about a month of staying with the couple in their home, my dad's wife decided it was best to take him to a facility where they could offer a physical therapy program while taking care of his other needs.

After a few weeks in that facility, Neill and I went by on a Sunday afternoon and took to Dad his usual Popeye's Chicken. He barely ate, and he was saying some pretty strange things. I was really concerned, so we called the nurse to come check on him. It turned out that his oxygen level was really low, so they called for an ambulance.

Once we got him to the hospital they found that he had double pneumonia. My dad never left critical care and passed away ten days after arriving there. That was the hardest ten days I had ever endured.

Dad had reserved his grave plot years earlier in his hometown of Baskin, Louisiana, right next to his father and mother, Bud and Inez Cupit. That is where we laid him to rest a few days after his passing.

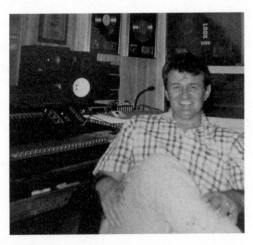

My dad, Jerry Cupit

The doors of that old country church where I grew up were overflowing with friends and family the day of his funeral. I wrote a eulogy to read that day but decided to let my godfather, Nolen Cowart, read it. I wasn't sure I could get through it without breaking down.

My daddy—you were the strongest man I've ever known! When I was a little girl you chased away the monsters in the middle of the night and stayed in my room until I fell back to sleep. I thought you could beat up anyone if I needed you to, and that was probably true!

I also thought you were the coolest dad in the world! After all, whose dad could play several instruments, karate chop a brick in half, build a house, run your own business, and tell a joke like no other! As far as I was concerned there was no better daddy!

You taught me so many things in this life—my first chords on guitar, how to write a song, the ins and outs of the music business, how to treat people, how to be strong, how to be my own unique person, how to go after what I wanted, how to have faith, and so, so much more.

As I got older, you and I grew even closer through the years making music together. We shared the crazy world of the music business—frequently complaining, sometimes laughing, sometimes crying, but always dreaming. We had our ups and downs along the way like most families, but our love never, ever wavered. Music was one connection, but it's love that binds us together forever.

When you got sick, Dad, I had never seen another person fight so hard to overcome such huge obstacles. You fought a strong, courageous fight for two years, but one human body can only endure so much.

I know you are in heaven now with no more pain and no more suffering to endure. You are perfect in every way, and I'm sure you're playing the guitar like never before, talking with Papaw Bud and Granny Ashley, and laughing with Snooky.

It gives me peace in knowing I can see you again one day to write another song and sing it with a choir of angels. I love you Daddy! You are my hero!

—Memarie

SEASON OF LIFE LESSON

That was by far the hardest season of life I had faced. Watching my dad lose his body, his pride, and his life in the most horrific way was almost unbearable. The ten days he was in critical care was nothing short of a terrible nightmare. Looking back now, it is even hard to type the words of the experience. But with every storm there is a lesson if we look deeply enough.

A few minutes before they intubated my dad with a breathing tube, I told him over and over how much I loved him. I also told him that every chance I had in the months leading up to that day. I am so thankful I was able to rebuild my relationship with him and we were able spend time together.

Never take for granted the time you have with anyone here on this earth. If there are fences that need rebuilding or words that need to be spoken, don't wait another second. I never imagined my dad's life would end at sixty-one years old.

As Dad slipped away to be with Jesus, I read him these words from the Bible:

The Lord is my shepherd; I shall not want. He maketh me to lie down in green pastures: he leadeth me beside the still waters. He restoreth my soul: he leadeth me in the paths of righteousness for his name's sake. Yea, though I walk through the valley of the shadow of death, I will fear no evil: for thou art with me; thy rod and thy staff they comfort me. Thou preparest a table before me in the presence of mine enemies: thou anointest my head with oil; my cup runneth over. Surely goodness and mercy shall follow me all the days of my life: and I will dwell in the house of the Lord forever. (Psalm 23 KJV)

I am thankful that I set aside my own pride in order to nurture my relationship with Dad. Thank you, God, for guiding my steps.

A man's pride shall bring him low: but honour shall uphold the humble in spirit. (Proverbs 29:23 KJV)

Honour thy father and thy mother: that thy days may be long upon the land which the lord thy God giveth thee. (Exodus 20:12 KJV)

CHAPTER 9

God Be with Me

2014 ended up being one of the most eventful years of my life—a year of both the best times and the worst times.

I decided the best way to relate this part of my journey was with my actual blog postings that I wrote during that season of life.

My longtime friend, Natasha (who is like a sister to me), encouraged me to blog during that difficult time, and I am so thankful I did. It not only helped me express my feelings throughout that season, but I received many e-mail messages from others telling me it helped them as well.

FAITH OVER FEAR BLOG

God Remains—10/11/2014

I debated many days about whether I wanted to share this on my blog. I am a private person, but I also thrive on using my experiences to help others. After much prayer I have decided to share some of my experiences over the last month in hope it will help someone else.

August 31, 2014 was the beginning of a whirlwind that is still spinning. That was the day my husband and I took my dad to the ER and found out he had double pneumonia. We lost my dad September 10. It was the hardest day I have gone through in this life. My dad will forever be in my memory and forever run through my veins. I will never know another man like him.

The love of a daughter and her daddy is something that can never be replaced. I think of him every day and realize this is something you never get over, but you learn to live with it. The loss is something I carry with me always, but with God helping me every step, I know I can walk with a lighter load.

Two days after returning to Nashville from my dad's memorial, I found out there was a possibility I had ovarian cancer and could not birth children. The loss of the possibility of having children very quickly turned into the need to heal my body. The doctor told me I needed immediate surgery.

I had my surgery seven days later, and I found out then that it was indeed ovarian cancer. I do not know what the future holds for me, but I do know that God will be with me. God is giving me a peace in the middle of this whirlwind around me. My dad taught me to be strong, and I am going to use all that strength to get through this bump in the road.

Every day, God shows me little signs of His presence.

Surviving Ovarian Cancer—10/17/2014

This has been a week of many emotions ranging from denial to peace, to anger, confusion, and back again to peace. You never think you are going to be diagnosed with ovarian cancer—or any type of cancer for that matter. I guess nobody does. But here I am.

My greatest sadness is the burden this puts on the ones I love. I like to be the one helping and supporting everyone around me, and this scenario does not fit into my usual scheme of things. Shock is the first response, and for me that quickly turned into *fix it mode*.

Once I got over the fact that I cannot fix it, I went to gathering all the information I could on ovarian cancer. Somehow this helps me regain a little more control over myself. At the end of the day, prayer is what saves me from my own thoughts and emotions. God is my constant, and I know He will get me through this with a victory!

I now know I have two different types of cancer. One was found in my ovaries and the other in my uterus. Surgery went well—with the removal of my ovaries, uterus, and fallopian tubes. My gynecologic oncologist also removed fluid found in my abdomen along with a couple of cancer cells. Chemotherapy is the next recommendation for my treatment to make sure that any possibly unseen cancer cells can, hopefully, be eradicated.

As we know, chemotherapy is a toxin, and it does kill good cells as well. There are also risks in damaging other organs through chemo. I am researching alternative methods that do not cause any harmful side effects in addition to researching chemotherapy. When something like this happens, the need for information is overwhelming.

I will continue to pray that God will lead me in the direction He wants me to go for my future cancer treatment. I am also open to any comments from other ovarian cancer survivors. Experience offers the best advice. God Bless!

The Road Ahead—10/21/2014

Today I met with my gynecologic oncologist. I have full confidence in her, her care, and her capabilities. I get a feeling that she really cares about me, and she is fully dedicated to what she does.

I have really struggled with the thought of chemotherapy over the last couple of weeks since my surgery. It has been a sea of emotion to say the least. Basically, what it comes down to now is me having the confidence in chemotherapy to cure my cancer.

I feel confident that it is the best source of treatment that I have at my disposal at this time. I do feel that with clinical trials on the horizon there will be more efficient drugs down the line. I also feel that prevention is the best method.

I plan on getting on a super-charged nutrition plan once chemotherapy is over, in order to make sure my immune system is working at its optimal level to keep cancer from recurring. I have basically been a healthy person my whole life—eating a balanced diet and exercising—but my downfall has always been sugar.

I have recently learned that sugar really does feed cancer. I am currently cutting back my sugar intake, and I encourage anyone reading this to do the same. Sugar causes inflammation in the body, and cancer is a type of inflammation. Sugar also aggravates or contributes to other diseases.

I'm sure chemotherapy is not going to be a walk in the park, but I know I will get through it. All of my organs are healthy and strong, which gives me a positive outlook for being cured. I know God led me to that fertility clinic in order for me to catch this early. I thought I was going to gain help that day for having children, but now I know that visit was to save my life.

God is in control, and He has a plan.

Please, please ladies, have your OBGYN do a blood test on you to check your CA125 levels, which is a cancer marker. A regular checkup does not detect it. Symptoms for ovarian cancer are almost non-existent until it's too late.

I caught this early, which was a miracle. I had no symptoms at all, but some of the symptoms are bloating, constipation, painful sex, frequent urination, and increased abdominal girth. As you see, these symptoms are not very unusual. It's best to go ahead and have your blood checked to be safe, especially if you have any type of cancer whatsoever in your family tree.

The road ahead is not going to be easy, but I know God will be walking right there beside me. My faith is not shaken, and my will is strong!

Keep Calm and Fight Cancer!—11/07/2014

Well I made it through my first two days of chemotherapy! I have to admit I was super nervous on Monday prior to the infusion. As I've talked about before, the thought of the chemotherapy drug running through my veins is a bit scary to me. I said a prayer before infusion, took a deep breath, and I was fine.

Monday was my *Taxol* day, which was given through IV. I'm a little nervous with IVs because I have fairly small veins, and at times nurses have had some trouble hitting my vein on the first try. I had a great IV nurse Monday, and she got it straight away. Sheeeeew—sigh of relief from me!

The nurse administered anti-nausea meds and fluids prior to the chemo to hopefully counteract any side effects. I tolerated the Taxol chemo very well and only felt tired afterward. That whole process took about five hours.

Yesterday was my IP[5] chemo day. That consisted of fluids given through IV for about two hours, which did take the nurse two tries for the vein. ICKY! But I was fine! Next, I was given more fluids through my IP port, which has a tube that travels straight to my abdominal cavity.

Once the fluids were in, she started to administer the chemo drug, *Cisplatin*. This drug is much harsher than the *Taxol* and causes more side effects, so I was geared up in *GI Jane* mode yesterday. That took about three hours, and once it is done you feel like a stuffed turkey, literally. My stomach was so swollen I could barely sit up and move about. It causes a little shortness of breath because there is so much fluid in your belly it pushes on your diaphragm causing breathing to be a little difficult.

Once they filled me with the *Cisplatin*, they turned me over to one side for fifteen minutes, then the other side for fifteen minutes, then the bed tilted my head down for fifteen minutes, and then, last, feet down for fifteen minutes. That was done twice for two hours total. Then I was finished—and soooo ready to go home!

The whole day lasted about nine hours. I waddled out of the hospital like a turkey, and I was pretty tired once I got home. Luckily by today my abdomen has absorbed most of the fluid, and the swelling has gone down. I'm just achy, like with the flu, and my belly hurts a bit, but I'm staying strong. I'm going to go down to my jewelry studio and try to get some new pieces made for the holidays to get my mind off feeling a little sick.

Mind over matter!

It is still early in this journey, but I'm just taking it one day at a time. If there is someone reading this who was just diagnosed with cancer or knows someone who was, I hope this blog will

---

5 IP—Intraperitoneal. https://en.wikipedia.org/wiki/Intraperitoneal_injection

help with your journey. I know it helped me to talk to others who had experienced it. Knowing some of the details of the experience makes it less scary.

My number one source of strength is my faith. I know God is with me through this journey. I am in constant talks with Him every day, and it offers much comfort. God promises to walk with us through this life of trials and heartache. He is in control, and He has a plan for me through this! I know it!

Jesus suffered for our sins on the cross so we could have eternal life with Him. In this life there is suffering, but in the next, if we follow Jesus it will be better than our human minds can even comprehend! But for now, I know I still have a purpose in this life, and that's why I know I'm going to beat this evil disease called cancer!

Beach and Blessings—11/20/2014

Today is a good day because this week is *chemo-free week*. Neill and I just arrived at the beach for an early Thanksgiving with family. One thing cancer does is make you appreciate the good days more than ever. Each day is a gift from God, and I am thankful for each one.

Last week was a challenging week to say the least. After my third round of chemotherapy (*Taxol*), I was having chest tightness and little twinges of pain for two days. My doctor sent me to the ER, where they found I had an irregular heartbeat and was low on a couple of nutrients. After giving me a round of magnesium and potassium I was sent home.

The next day I had an appointment with a cardiologist for further evaluation to find out if the chemo has affected my heart. Between him and my oncologist I am hoping they can figure it out soon. Another possibility is that just sheer anxiety is causing the chest issues. The cardiologist feels there is nothing to worry about, and my heart is not damaged.

This week off chemotherapy has been a blessing! I was able to sing at church Wednesday night with some great people and enjoy using my voice to serve God. It was wonderful therapy for me. God is good! I'm hoping I can continue to sing some throughout my chemotherapy journey, as long as I'm feeling up to it.

It is one day at a time, and I have to remind myself of that. Some days I can function pretty well, but other days I have to listen to my body and let it rest. Tonight, I will be shaving my head and drawing strength from my inner *GI Jane*. I loved having my long hair, but it is just hair. Putting it in perspective, I am glad I am here to get to shave my head. It will grow back, and I now have an excuse to buy more fabulous hats—ha-ha-ha.

For the next few days I'm going to rest, relax, rejuvenate, count my blessings, and enjoy the beautiful sunsets on the beach. Thanking God for this time to enjoy life!

Back on the Juice—Chemo, that is!—12/05/2014

So, I'm back on the juice today (chemo, that is). I was off for two weeks because I needed more tests done on my heart. The MRI was clear and fine. I do have some cardiac arrhythmia, which they will keep an eye on. I'm hoping this is something that will go away after chemotherapy is over. Other than that, I'm doing well.

Speaking of juice, I've been juicing every day—making sure not to use any raw veggies and washing my fruit with antibacterial soap, then peeling it before blending. Any veggies I use have to be cooked while on chemo, so I cook my kale and spinach, then freeze. This works great!

My go-to juice recipe:

- One cup of kale
- A few apple slices
- Ginger root (just a small thumbnail size)
- Half an orange
- A few slices of frozen melon
- A few cucumber slices
- Put all of the ingredients into a *NutriBullet*, fill it with water, and blend.

I'm also drinking tons of water each day with lemon. Lemon is a natural detox, and the Lord knows this chemo is toxic. The lemon helps to flush it out. Chemotherapy also tends to dehydrate you, so drinking more water than ever in your life is key. So far, no dehydration for me! I know it's from all the water I drink daily.

I also eat small bits of food every two to three hours instead of three big meals a day. This has helped so much with nausea. It sounds weird, but it's true! I keep either crackers or a banana by my bedside every night, because when I wake in the morning I'm nauseous, and this helps a lot.

I do stretch every day, which helps with the muscle soreness and tightness. I also just started taking baths every night with Epsom salt and baking soda added to the bath water—a great detox for lymph nodes, and also great for muscle soreness. I use this as my time to pray and meditate. Everyone needs to do this, especially cancer patients.

Calming your mind is the best thing for your spirit and body. I've cut out *dairy* for the weeks I'm on chemo because lots of chemotherapy patients become lactose intolerant. I decided to not take the chance. On my week off, I have some dairy. I also cut out red meat and sugar during my chemo weeks. These are also hard to digest, and digestion is always a problem during chemotherapy. Besides, both are just hard on your body, period.

I do have some if I want on my off-week. A girl has got to have some pleasure during this unpleasant time. I hope this helps anyone who might be just finding out they need chemo, or someone who has a loved one about to begin it. God is good! I'm enjoying my good times and embracing the not-so-good.

Staying strong in the storm!

I'm also wigging it out—wearing a wig, that is, ha-ha! I'm not stressing over the hair loss as much as I thought I would. Again, God is good! I truly believe He has helped me with this and relieved me of this unnecessary burden and worry. I've been trying out new hairstyles and making it fun!

A Thankful Christmas—12/25/2014

Today on Christmas, I am so thankful for two rounds of treatments down and only three to go, which leaves a total of nine treatments.

I was so relieved that my second round was much easier on me than the first. My oncologist prescribed me magnesium and potassium supplements, which seem to have helped with some of the side effects. The heart problems I had on the first round were gone for the second round of treatments. I'm praying I have the same results for the next three rounds.

I also feel that the Epsom salt baths have helped to lessen the side effects, as they are a natural detox. Last week I started reading a book by Gloria Copeland called *And Jesus Healed Them All*. I would recommend this to anyone needing healing in his or her life. It helps to get your mind right when it comes to faith and healing.

I am now thanking God for the healing He is doing in my body now and in the future. Even if I do not feel it or see it some days, I am thanking Him because I am expecting healing, not just hoping for it.

Just a few months before I was diagnosed with ovarian cancer, my family doctor diagnosed me with *Raynaud's Syndrome*. I started having symptoms of that during last summer. If I got the slightest bit cold, my fingers got numb, tingly, and got splotchy white spots on them. That also happened to my toes, which could be painful at times.

I told my oncologist about that, and she did not know of Raynaud's having a connection with cancer. I felt like once the cancer was out of my body it would go away. She just said it would be interesting to see what happens. I really do not think she felt it would have any effect on it. But miraculously after the operation, I haven't had a Raynaud's episode to this day. My oncologist can't explain it.

I know without a doubt that God is working in my body to heal me. Like I said, I am now expecting healing, not hoping for it. This unexplained healing is already proof enough for me. Thank you, God, on this Christmas Day, for all your blessings.

New Year's Resolution: *Journey Back to the Soul*—01/02/2015

At 4:00 a.m. on December 31st, my birthday, I couldn't sleep, so I began to pray and thank God for the great news I had been given the day before. My CA125 (cancer marker) count was down to eight, and anything below thirty is good.

As I was praying—and honestly, dozing off and waking up—I started thinking about a book that I've been wanting to write for a few years now. I started working on it off and on in 2014, but not with a real focus.

I knew I wanted it to be an autobiography of sorts, but not where the focus is just on me. I wanted it to relate the lessons learned and the insights gained through experiences, mistakes, ups, downs, and so forth. And I wanted it to show how these things are all wrapped up in the loving guidance of my Creator, who has always been with me on my personal journey since birth.

Between 4:00 a.m. and 6:00 a.m. God gave me the title, *Journey Back to the Soul*, and many other insights that have given me a real focus for this book. I decided to blog about it, so I can have accountability for this from friends and family. We all need that, right?

With my recent health issues, it has made me realize when you want to accomplish something you can't wait even one more day. You have to do it now, because we really do not know what tomorrow will bring. I am asking God to bless this book. I pray for His will to shine through it, and that it will be done.

My hope is that by reading about my journey back to *my* soul, it will inspire others to begin or push forward in continuing their own journeys back to *their* souls. Have a blessed 2015 everyone!

[Side note: Well, it took a little longer than I thought when I wrote this blog post, but thank you, Jesus, I finally did it! Some goals take longer than anticipated, but that's okay as long as you keep moving forward to fruition.]

Change Your Perspective; Change Your Outcome—01/25/2015

I am now in the middle of my fourth cycle of treatments. I have one more treatment on Monday, and this wraps the fourth of six cycles. I'm so excited to say I'm finally over the hump!

Somewhere in the middle of this cycle I began to think of my original thoughts about the chemotherapy itself. I worried about how it might injure my healthy cells and organs. Then about halfway through, I began to look at it as a healing process I have to go through in order to allow God to eradicate the cancer cells.

Now in coming over the mountain of this process, I know that my cancer markers are dropping, and healing is taking place! My perspective has changed. Now I see it as a sort of cleansing process for my body in order for God to prepare me for the next stage of my life's journey.

A few years ago I felt a stirring of the Spirit of God like I had never felt before. It came at a time when I felt I had no one to turn to. Through God I was given the strength to get out of a difficult situation. I became stronger because of it. I learned that if I put all my faith in God, victory could be won!

2013 became one of the best years of my life. So many doors were open to me as I prayed each day for God to lead me every step of the way. 2014 rounded out as a year I will never forget for so many reasons. It was filled with the best times, and the worst times, but through it all God was always there by my side.

What I learned in 2014 is that God never gives you anything for which He doesn't prepare you. Which brings me back to my change in perspective on my chemotherapy treatments.

I know that when our bodies are stressed mentally and emotionally, the stress will manifest itself physically as well. Many of these stresses we put on ourselves. They pile up and pile up over the years. That's not to say that I gave myself cancer, because I do not believe that.

There are so many factors that play into that, and I am not a doctor, so I can't self-diagnose. What I can do is look at these treatments as a way for my body to cleanse itself back to ground zero. I feel I have been doing that emotionally and spiritually over the last few years.

Now it's time to cleanse my body of this cancer that has been growing without me even knowing it. My emotional and spiritual cleansing has come from forgiveness, faith, love, trust, and discipline. Now my body is catching up, and it's time to cleanse.

It may sound weird, but for me it makes complete sense. It's a perspective that gives this treatment a purpose. When you have a purpose, everything else changes for the better. So, cleansing it is! Mid-March will be the end of the cleansing, and boy, will I be a happy camper when this cleanse is a wrap!

Chemotherapy and Me—03/19/2015

I finished up my last chemotherapy treatment last week. I can't explain the weight that has been lifted. You can talk to other people who have been through it. But until you experience it for yourself, you really do not understand.

I wanted to share with everyone a few unknowns that I learned through the journey of chemotherapy in hopes of helping prepare others who may have to go through it. I can really only speak to those who will undergo ovarian cancer treatment. There are some similarities in various chemotherapy drugs, but some of the side effects are different. So in that respect, I can only tell you what I experienced with my IP and IV treatments for ovarian/uterine cancer.

One of the things that I did not anticipate was all of the odd things that happen in your body. Everything basically is out of whack. You have unexplained aches and pains throughout your body—muscle aches and also pockets of soreness under your skin in various places, all over your body, at different times. I came to realize this was the toxin getting trapped and trying to move through my system.

The thing that helped with that the most was my Epsom salt and baking soda baths every day. If I had a lot of soreness, I would take two a day some days. Get ready—this will make you sweat, but it's the best thing for you.

The IP therapy fills your abdomen with the chemotherapy drug and also an additional liter of fluids. For the first treatment I took all the fluids but soon found out this was too much for me. I was so full that the pressure was too much on my chest and heart. My oncologist ordered to have the additional fluid left out.

I would say that if you were feeling any pressure on your chest or shortness of breath on your first treatment, let your oncologist know ASAP. They will either cut the additional fluid out completely or cut it in half.

After my third treatment I experienced unexplained heart racing, chest tightness, and even pain. Some of the chemotherapy drugs do tend to make your heart race and even raise your blood pressure. If you ever feel any tightness or pain in your chest call your doctor ASAP! I had to make an emergency room visit and found out I was low on potassium and also magnesium. My oncologist resolved this by having me take supplements throughout the remainder of my treatment, and I was fine.

I almost left this one out because it is extremely rare, but I feel I need to continue with open honesty: On my last treatment of *Cisplatin* chemotherapy through my IP port, I had an anaphylactic reaction. I was fine for all my other previous treatments, but evidently I built up an allergy to this drug.

Apparently, this has been documented in the medical books for this particular drug—when given through IP—only one other time. My first symptom was a runny nose and itchy eyes. If this happens during chemotherapy, buzz the nurse immediately. I did not, because I thought it was seasonal allergies.

When my lips began to swell, I buzzed the nurse. My throat and tongue started to swell very quickly after that. The nurses were on top of it. They got it under control to stop the reaction before it got worse. My takeaway from this is that you must call the nurse if you have any change at all in your body during treatment. It could save your life!

Another obstacle I did not anticipate was all the fluid your body retains, and the weight gain. You always hear of people losing weight through chemotherapy treatment. I had never heard of weight gain. I believe that for some people who have a more advanced cancer, they lose weight because of the cancer itself, not the chemotherapy.

Don't get me wrong. There are some who lose weight if they get extremely sick from nausea and so forth.

My therapy included a high dose of steroids, which of course puffs you up and can make you gain weight. My oncologist said it's better to gain than to lose because you want your body to remain strong to fight. If you lose even a few pounds it weakens you and can cause you to miss some of your treatments.

Your goal is to not to miss any treatments! Needless to say, she was happy with my weight gain. Me? not so much! Hah. In saying this, I will recommend that you should eat every three hours during your treatment weeks.

When you are nauseous, the last thing you want to do is eat. I found if I forced myself to eat every three hours it helped with the nausea. When you are taking the chemo drugs it tends to cause lots of acid in your stomach, and keeping something in it helps a lot. Even if it's just to eat a few crackers, you need to force yourself. Like my doctor said, it is better to gain than lose.

If you get in the habit of not eating just because you feel nauseous, you will lose weight—because you are nauseous a lot. Take my word and eat.

One of my *go-tos* was my protein Juice Plus+® Complete shakes.[6] When I could not eat anything else, I could still drink a shake. I completely lost my appetite for meat—especially red meat. Peanut butter became my best friend for protein. If nothing else, peanut butter with crackers and Juice Plus+® Complete shakes will get you through those rough days.

Lymphedema[7] was another bump in the road that I was not prepared for. The doctors do not really talk about this to you. I understand they are focused on treating the cancer. There is a lot on their plate just concentrating on that. But if you have any type of cancer treatment—surgery, chemotherapy, or radiation—then you are at a significant risk for lymphedema, unfortunately.

The key is treating it early when you see the first signs of it. Lymphedema is when the lymph nodes get overloaded and can't filter well. Our lymphatic system[8] is like our body's personal vacuum cleaner. It filters toxins, waste, and so forth out of our system.

When I had my surgery, my oncologist took out lymph nodes to test for cancer—leaving me with less than the good Lord gave

---

6   Juice Plus+® is a company that specializes in natural nourishment products.
7   https://www.mayoclinic.org/diseases-conditions/lymphedema/ symptoms-causes/syc-20374682
8   https://www.livescience.com/26983-lymphatic-system.html

me. Of course, the body has to work harder in those areas to filter out the toxins.

My lymph nodes were taken from my pelvic area, putting me at risk for lymphedema in my legs. Lots of breast cancer patients get lymphedema in their arms. Mine is in my right leg. I will get swelling in my leg if I'm on my feet a lot, especially standing in one spot.

I'm currently getting lymphatic drainage massage, which helps. If I had known to look for this condition from the beginning, I would have started the massage earlier to hopefully prevent it. I would recommend anyone going through cancer treatment to keep a close eye on the limbs that could be affected. Look for the slightest swelling, so you can jump on treating it early.

This is considered a lifelong condition with no cure—only maintenance—so do not let it go untreated. I believe I will get my lymphedema under control. God will help me through this just like He did with the cancer. I caught it fairly early, so I am keeping the faith that it will be reversible.

I hope this blog will help anyone going through cancer treatment. It gives you a heads-up on a few things that you do not hear talked about very often but can surely affect you. *Mind over body* is the biggest, most powerful component of your cancer treatment process. Through the stripes of Jesus on the cross, we are healed.[9]

Believe this and make it your truth! God wants us to be healthy and be warriors for Him!

---

9 "But He was wounded for our transgressions, He was bruised for our iniquities; the chastisement for our peace was upon Him, and by His stripes we are healed" (Isaiah 53:5).

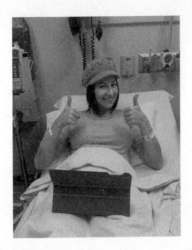

Chemo days

Radiation Therapy and Staying Strong—04/27/2015

I haven't blogged in a while, so I decided to bring everyone up to date. I started my radiation therapy a week ago. I will be finished by the end of this week. They took me into surgery to remove my port that was used for my chemotherapy. The doctor then put a sleeve in my cervix in order to help with the radiation therapy. They are administering brachytherapy radiation.

Instead of going into detail, you can look this up if interested— ha, ha. It's not your typical radiation therapy. The good news is that it targets directly where it is needed, which is my cervix. Because a bit of cancer was found in my uterus, the radiologist wanted to zap my cervix to kill any microscopic cancer cells that might not have been seen in the initial surgery.

The days I go for radiation are not fun, but at least all my other days in between are good. I will cross the finish line this Friday! There is a mix of emotions that comes with the end of my therapy. I will say that I was warned by others who have gone through this journey that fears creep in either toward the end of therapy or when it's over.

Once they are not actively fighting the cancer, many survivors are left feeling helpless. I did not expect to feel this because I've really had a positive outlook on this battle I'm fighting. I was surprised when the feelings crept in once I finished the chemotherapy. I had a couple of days following chemotherapy where I felt like, "Now what?"

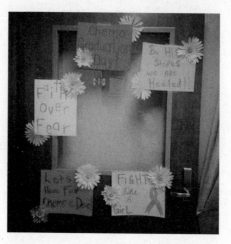

My mom helped me decorate my infusion-room door
to celebrate my last chemo treatment.

When your whole life revolves around fighting it for seven or eight months, you feel helpless when you are not actively fighting it anymore. It was comforting to know that this feeling is natural for us survivors. That is why I am mentioning it now.

I prayed my way through it. God did take away the fears. It is possible I might feel a little fear come back after I wrap up my last treatment of radiation Friday, but I'm praying I will not. Now I know I have to trust God more than ever and put my faith in Him. When all the doctor's work is done and I go back to life as usual, I will put trust in God to keep me strong and fight this fight for me.

These are the times that test your faith. It also makes your faith stronger when you let go and trust in Him. My prayer is that God will take the lead more than ever before in my life and take me where He wants me to go. My hope is that my struggles will be a testament to others—they will be a help to others in knowing God is always there, even in our hardest times.

We can trust and lean on the Word of God and know that He can make all things work for His good.[10]

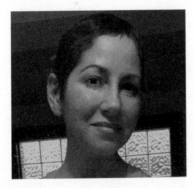

This was the day I decided to ditch the wig.
My treatments were over, and my hair was growing
back just a little. Yay! I'm no longer bald!

My Top Ten List—05/22/2015
(what I learned through my ovarian cancer journey)

I decided that in light of David Letterman's retirement I would do my own top ten list. Some are funny, and some serious. So here it goes:

---

10 "And we know that in all things God works for the good of those who love him, who have been called according to his purpose" (Romans 8:28).

TOP TEN THINGS I LEARNED FROM
MY JOURNEY WITH OVARIAN CANCER

1. I don't like being bald.
2. Chemotherapy is no joke.
3. If you find yourself saying, "*one day* I'm going to do this or that," why wait? Do it now while you're healthy, because time flies too fast.
4. If you need to say anything to anyone, don't wait another day. Say it today.
5. Don't stress over the small stuff. I'm too blessed to be depressed!
6. Give thanks to God—even in your darkest hours. In return He brings you peace in your situation.
7. Tell the people you love that you love them anytime, anywhere.
8. You are stronger than you think.
9. Create your own happiness every day. Even the smallest things can bring a smile.
10. Chemo-brain can make you forget you're bald sometimes— when you are wearing a wig.

My Post-chemotherapy Journey Part 1—07/06/2015

I will start out by saying that I am so thankful to be alive and be cancer free. Without my faith in God, and without the wonderful doctors and nurses, I would not be here today. I have decided to blog about my continued journey, because as I'm finding out, the journey isn't over.

A lot of people think that once treatments are complete the survivor's fight is over. This is a large misconception. This was my own misconception—as it is for most survivors. I want to document this side of cancer survivorship in order to hopefully prepare other survivors. I hope it also helps their families and friends understand them better.

I will start with the emotional side of post-treatment.

Once I was finished, I had a surge of relief. I was so thankful—and I still am—to be finished with chemotherapy and radiation. I very quickly started feeling like my old self and started regaining energy. Another survivor warned me that I might have an onset of post-treatment depression, but I was certain I would not. To my surprise, she was right.

About two weeks later, I had feelings of, "what now?" When you're not aggressively fighting the cancer, you feel a little helpless and more vulnerable. I had to put my faith completely in God once again and let Him carry me through it. That feeling only lasted a couple of days as I turned it all over to God. As I draw closer to God, my fear goes away.

The relationships I am building at my church home are a huge part of my recovery. It feels incredible to be a part of something bigger than yourself. Coming together with other believers who are passionate about Jesus is so important to me, especially in the times in which we live. Using my God-given gift of music has never been more rewarding!

On the physical side of things, chemotherapy and radiation really wreaked havoc on my body. Again, I will say, I'm thankful that we have treatments that can now cure some cancers. I'm thankful that I'm cancer free. Now I just have to pray that in time these side effects will go away. I'm dealing with neuropathy in my hands and feet, lymphedema in my right leg, arthritis symptoms, immediate menopause symptoms. and the dreaded *chemo-brain* (it's real).

In my next blog I will go into more detail on each of these. The neuropathy came on about a month after chemotherapy was complete and continued to get worse for weeks, and then leveled off. I am happy to say now, after three months, it is somewhat better. I'm hoping it will continue to get better with time. I am taking a vitamin B complex to help with this.

Tomorrow I have my first office appointment at a place called *Internal Balance* in Brentwood, Tennessee. The owner, Tamara, is a biochemist and nutritionist who has developed a DNA testing program to detox and rebuild the body in a natural way. Another ovarian cancer survivor referred me to her.

For those of you who know me well, you know I'm a naturalist and prefer to help my body heal itself whenever possible. My initial conversation with Tamara was amazing! I really feel that God led me to her. She incorporates her strong Christian beliefs into her practice, which I appreciate greatly. In our first conversation she gave me a Scripture to read out loud every day. She told me that this is a very healing Scripture.

When I got off the phone with her, I was praying and hoping God had led me to her for help in cleansing my body and continuing my healing process. I looked at the paper where I had written the Bible verse, Matthew 4:10.

I opened my Bible app on my iPhone, and as I went to hit the search icon I happened to notice that Matthew was already open, and to my shock it was open to Matthew 4:10. I started crying so hard and thanking God for this sign and for this word He had given me to fight the enemy with.

For me the enemy was cancer, and now, physical pains. This is the verse I read out loud and have continued to read out loud every day since:

Jesus said to him, "Away from me Satan! For it is written: 'Worship the Lord your God and serve him only.'" Then the devil left him, and angels came and attended him. (Matthew 4:10-11)

When we speak God's Word out loud, it is so powerful! I believe this with all my heart.

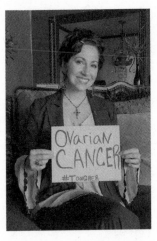

Grow through what you go through.

My Post-chemotherapy Journey Part 2—08/18/2015 (Is your beauty bag toxic?)

I wanted to share with you a few things I have learned about skin and beauty products over the last few years. It's amazing how God was already leading me to educate myself about these things even before I knew I had cancer. As I've already told you, I have always been a naturalist, and the fact I was putting things on my skin that could be harmful was appalling. I discovered that Europe banned 1,373 chemicals from cosmetic products while the USA had only banned 8. That's right, only 8! Basically, the FDA turns a blind eye to the beauty industry. I will say it is slowly getting better.

TOP INGREDIENTS I RECOMMEND YOU AVOID:

- PARABENS—Get these out of your life! The good news is that you can now find many products that do not contain parabens but instead use other healthier ingredients to replace them. Look at your hair product, lotions, and makeup ingredient list closely.
- PARFUM—This is a fancy way of saying "fragrance." It can cause asthma, acne, and allergies.
- FORMALDEHYDE—It prevents bacteria growth and can cause cancer.
- TOLUENE—This is a super-strong solvent used to dissolve paint. Toluene is found in many popular nail polishes—not good!
- COAL TAR DYES—Colors are listed as "CI"[11] followed by a five-digit number or called out by color name and number. For example, if you see something like, "Blue 1" or "FD&C Blue No. 1," run.

One of the major changes I have made in my skincare routine is cutting out parabens. Numerous studies have shown that parabens are directly linked to cancer—specifically breast cancer because it will mimic estrogen. The only moisturizer I use on my body is organic, virgin coconut oil.

I buy mine at the grocery store. This was an easy, economical switch that anyone can make. It's actually cheaper than buying body lotion at expensive beauty spas and much better for your skin. Research coconut oil yourself and discover all the wonderful benefits!

---

11 CI is the abbreviation for "Color Index."

Another change I made in my skin-care routine was to make my own face cream and eye cream. The face cream I make fights wrinkles, and it also calms sensitive skin. The eye cream moisturizes and also helps with dark circles and puffiness. It feels good to know I am no longer putting harsh chemicals on my body.

SIMPLE DIY EYE CREAM

- 1/2 cup organic extra virgin coconut oil
- 6 vitamin E capsules

Microwave the Coconut oil for 10 seconds then add the Vitamin E by pricking the capsules with a pin and extracting the oil. Mix together with a toothpick, pour into a small glass container with lid and refrigerate for a couple of hours.

This will last a long time because a little goes a long way. But since this does not contain any preservatives, it will not last as long as over-the-counter creams. It will last about two months unused, so don't make more than you can use.

DIY FACE CREAM

- 3/4 cup organic extra virgin coconut oil
- 1 tablespoon of aloe vera gel (get the purest stuff you can—I scrape it from my own plant).
- 4 drops of pure frankincense essential oil
- 4 drops of pure lavender essential oil

Add all ingredients in a blender (I use my *Magic Bullet*) and mix. Store it in an airtight glass container in a cool spot. Again, a little goes a long way and lasts about two months. Enjoy!

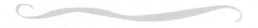

SEASON OF LIFE LESSON

That season of life taught me just how strong we really are as humans. When you have the Holy Spirit within you, the strength rises up as if you have a superhero inside of you. I won't say dealing with my ordeal wasn't hard, because it was the fight of my life. But I knew I was not walking the road alone.

I had angry moments, sad moments, and times I wanted to kick and scream. You never think you can handle anything like cancer until you face it. You either give up and let it take you over, both physically and emotionally, or you make a decision to fight. I made the decision to fight, and I'm so thankful I did!

Be strong and of a good courage, fear not, nor be afraid of them: for the Lord thy God, he it is that doth go with thee; he will not fail thee, nor forsake thee. (Deuteronomy 31:6 KJV)

He giveth power to the faint; and to them that have no might he increaseth strength. (Isaiah 40:29 KJV)

Let all that I am praise the Lord; may I never forget the good things he does for me. He forgives all my sins and heals all my diseases. (Psalms 103:2-3 NLT)

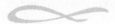

You can find my song, *God be with Me*, on iTunes or Spotify under *Memarie Gayle*.

CHAPTER 10

Fear and Victory

This chapter begins with another of my blog entries.

Ovarian Cancer Checkup—Fear and Victory!—09/26/2016

This week was a roller coaster of emotions for me. I'm almost sure no one else would have known this, although I did tell my husband. I never wanted my fears or concerns to burden anyone else. I always want to just be a light to others and not a downer. Sometimes this is harder than at other times, and this week was one of those times.

The week started out with my usual work of creating jewelry and brainstorming to grow my business. Wednesday started out great with a fitting at Levy's clothing in Green Hills. I appeared on News Channel 5, *Talk of the Town*, Thursday, so I needed to get fitted for the fall fashion I was going to wear. Two other survivors of ovarian cancer and I were modeling fall fashion to bring awareness to ovarian cancer.

Ironically, as soon as I left my fitting, I had to go straight to Vanderbilt Ingram Cancer Center for my checkup. When I arrived at Vanderbilt, I had to wait for a short time to get my blood drawn for my lab workups. For some reason fear crept in as I was getting my blood drawn. The needle went into my arm, and it really hurt that time! The nurse said I was probably a little dehydrated.

When she removed the needle, it hurt even more than the insertion. Ouchy! After I had my blood drawn, I returned to the lobby to wait for my gynecologic oncologist exam. I was there much longer than usual, and for the first time in a long time, fear was knocking. The pain of the needle prick seemed to bring back old memories—unlike any of my other checkups thus far.

September is *Ovarian Cancer Awareness Month,* so for this entire month it has been at the forefront of my mind. I keep thinking about the statistics, the negative outcomes, and the recurrences so many women face with this deadly disease. I'm over a year out from my surgery, completed chemotherapy, and radiation. It suddenly hit me that for many women it's between the one-year and two-year marks when ovarian cancer recurs.

I began to pray and rebuke those thoughts and fears. I went on to have my pelvic exam done by my gynecologic oncologist, and everything seemed good. Then I just had to wait on my CA125 blood test to come back. It wasn't until the next day that I received the results.

All my tests were good and showed nothing alarming. I had a small little cry of relief and immediately praised God for all He had done for me. Wow! how quickly we forget in our fast-paced lives just how far we have come. In that moment, I felt the gratitude and love for Christ rush over me.

Sometimes the knock of Satan on our door reminds us to always run to God in everything we face each day. This knock was my reminder. It tested my faith once again, but all in all, I came out of it in victory. Praise God from whom all blessings flow!

It wasn't until September of 2017 when I felt that same fear creeping back into my mind once again. In addition to my involvement with *Chic Awearness*,[12] I had just created a new jewelry collection with my friend and fellow ovarian cancer survivor, Leora, to bring awareness to the disease.

With ovarian cancer constantly at the forefront of my mind, I was once again finding myself a little anxious. That went on for about two weeks. One afternoon after delivering jewelry to a local boutique, I passed my church, as I often do when driving that route. But that time I felt a prompting to stop. Once I got in the parking lot, I said, "Okay God, here I am. Now what."

I felt led to go in and talk to Pastor Sandy, a remarkable woman of God whom I greatly respect. I didn't know if she would even be there, but I went in and asked for her anyway. She was indeed there. I sat down with her and began to tell her about the fear that was attacking me once again. Ovarian cancer statistics were swirling in my mind. It was causing me much anxiety.

She told me, "You are a healed child of God, and those statistics have nothing to do with you. This is a direct attack of Satan on your mind. You have to rebuke those thoughts and get serious about telling him to leave your mind. You have to fight those

12 *Chic Awearness* is an annual event held in Nashville, Tennessee, to raise awareness and funding for Ovarian Cancer research.

thoughts with the same strength you used to fight cancer and get through all your treatments."

"Get mad about it!" she said. "Speak Scripture out loud when those thoughts come to mind, and speak it with strength."

She then laid her hands on me and prayed a powerful prayer. I can say, in that moment I felt a lifting of the pressure that was on me. She also gave me a list of Scriptures to meditate on and use in those times when the enemy attacked my mind.

I walked out of there feeling a hundred percent better than when I walked into her office. I read the Scriptures. I let her words of wisdom sink into my mind over the next few days and reflected back on them for weeks after. Thank you, Jesus, for my church family and for your Word—my sword and shield.

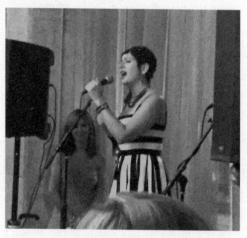

Singing & Speaking at Chic Awearness

SEASON OF LIFE LESSON

Never underestimate fear, and never underestimate the power of God to eradicate it! Fight it with the Word of God. Fight it with a vigor as if your life depended on it!

Fear and anxiety can be worse than physical illness at times. If you do not get it under the power of Jesus and rebuke it from your life, it can actually manifest into physical illness. Build your faith around yourself like a hedge—not letting fear build a gate to gain entry.

Use these Scriptures as I did, and allow the power of the Word to cleanse your life of fear and anxiety:

> *Do not be anxious about anything, but in everything by prayer and supplication with thanksgiving let your requests be made known to God. And the peace of God, which surpasses all understanding, will guard your hearts and your minds in Christ Jesus.*
>
> (Philippians 4:6-7 ESV)

> *Humble yourselves, therefore, under the mighty hand of God so that at the proper time he may exalt you, casting all your anxieties on him, because he cares for you.* (1 Peter 5:6-7 ESV)

> *Therefore do not worry about tomorrow, for tomorrow will worry about itself. Each day has enough trouble of its own.*
>
> (Matthew 6:34)

> *Anxiety weighs down the heart, but a kind word cheers it up.*
>
> (Proverbs 12:25)

> *A cheerful heart is good medicine, but a crushed spirit dries up the bones.* (Proverbs 17:22)

CHAPTER 11

New Hope New Life

As I write this chapter I am sitting in a hotel room in Houston. I was asked to speak at an ovarian cancer survivorship conference about the top concerns of survivorship. Since my diagnosis, I have been asked to speak and sing for several Christian women's conferences and ovarian cancer events. I've sung my entire life, but getting up and speaking is a different *ball game*.

I was the girl who avoided speech classes in high school and college at all cost. Looking back, maybe one speech class would have not been such a bad idea! But as I knew He would, Jesus carried me, and the event was very rewarding and such a blessing. What a way to come full circle—not only in conquering cancer but getting the opportunity to share my story of conquering fear with other survivors who share the same concerns.

Once you have heard the doctor say the word, "cancer," you are changed forever. It adds layers to your life that you never expected—good ones and not so good ones. But the truth is, none of us know how long we have left on this earth, so why waste valuable time worrying about the when, the why, and the how? I just want to live it, because all we truly have is the present.

I'm so grateful for the journey. The valleys and the mountains have so many lessons for us all. I promise you that God is working in every one of them. We just have to be awake and alert to the whisper of the Holy Spirit. I'm learning every day more and more how to hear His voice.

A few weeks ago as I was leaving church, I received a call from a church-friend. She asked if I was still there, and I told her I wasn't, but I could come back. I sensed in her voice that it was important, so I turned around and went back to the church to meet her.

She knew my husband and I had been on an adoption waiting list for two years since I had finished all my cancer treatments. She had met a young lady who desired to adopt out her child but didn't know how to go about it. Out of respect to the birth mom I will not go into all her reasons, but she was making the most loving yet hard decision of her lifetime.

My husband and I met her the next day, and we instantly felt at ease with each other. She just seemed to be a sweet girl in a bad situation. We came to an adoption agreement with her by the end of our three-hour meeting. We decided to go with her to her doctor's office for check-ups. We quickly began preparing for our new baby girl, who was due in three months. I jumped right in and completely opened my heart.

We had two baby showers, and I got the nursery decorated for our baby girl, Sevilla. We decided to name her after my and Neill's favorite city in Spain as well as our great grandmothers, who were both named Elizabeth. She would be Sevilla Elizabeth Jobe.

We were there in the room the day the birth mom was induced. I was at her bedside holding her hand throughout the entire birth. I had never experienced the miracle of life like that before. Tears were flowing, and our hearts were so full!

She was the most beautiful baby we had ever seen. Words cannot describe the joy we felt that day. The hospital gave us our own room to be with our baby girl *24/7*. We fed her and cared for her for two days and nights.

The birth mom came into our room before she was discharged. She told us how thankful she was that she had found us, and that we were going to give the baby such a wonderful, loving home. She said she knew she had made the right decision. That all made us feel secure with everything.

But later that afternoon our nurse walked into our room with a *deer-in-the-headlights* look and told us the birth mom had decided to keep the baby. She would be coming back to the hospital to get her later that day. Our hearts dropped! We were in complete shock. "How could she do this?" I thought to myself. "How could she string us along like this?"

We would not let ourselves believe it was happening. We held on to hope until there was no hope left. A couple of hours went by, and the nurse came back to say the birth mom was on her way to the hospital. We had to leave before she arrived. It was as if we had stepped into a horrible dream. It was an out-of-body experience I was having in that moment.

The baby's mother said we could have a few minutes with the baby to say our goodbyes. I kissed her little forehead and prayed for God to take care of her and watch over her. I loved her soooo much! Neill and I both did. She stole our hearts in such a short time. We left the hospital that day completely empty, confused, heartbroken, and angry.

The anger was overwhelming. It was something my husband and I had to work through over the next couple of months. We asked our adoption agency to take us off the Waiting Family list so we could mourn the loss of little Sevilla. We knew we were not ready to open our hearts to another child yet. I was so certain that God gave Sevilla to us that I had a hard time knowing how to reconcile my feelings.

As I worked through my emotions of anger, it gave way to hurt, then forgiveness, and finally to healing. I continued to pray and never let go of my faith. It was hard, but I knew if I could make it through cancer, I could make it through that loss. We may never know all the reasons why that happened until we see God face to face, but I believe in His will and His way.

One thing I do know is that I will continue to pray for Sevilla until my last breath. Maybe that was the reason, or at least one of the reasons God gave her to us for that short time. No one can ever have too many prayer warriors.

On the first of January we decided we were ready to go back on the waiting list for a baby. We also started looking at adopting a child from foster care. On Wednesday, the third of January, our adoption agency called us with a possible adoption match. We looked through the birth mom's and birth father's paperwork and decided to move forward.

We were afraid, but we also knew another child deserved our whole hearts just as much as Sevilla did.

At that time, the birth parents didn't know the sex of the child. The baby was due in two weeks, so we had to make a decision. We talked and prayed about it and on Friday wired the money to cover the adoption expenses.

By Friday night the agency got a call from the birth parents telling them we would have a baby girl. I was ecstatic! How perfect. We were already prepared for a girl! We had a closet full of clothes for her, and the nursery was all set for a *girly* girl.

But on Monday morning I found out just how much of a sense of humor God has. We got a call at 6:30 a.m. from the agency congratulating us on a baby boy. Wow! Wait! What? Yes, she said a baby *boy*! The nurse practitioner who made the decision earlier had obviously been mistaken.

We kicked it into high gear, booked a flight, and two hours later we were on a plane to Des Moines, Iowa. On the flight to Iowa, we decided to name him after both our late fathers—*James* after Neill's dad, and *Dean* after my dad. So, *James Dean Jobe* it was! I even made Neill shake on it. Ha, ha, ha!

I have to admit, our hearts were cautious, but we also knew that little baby boy deserved all of our heart—not half, not three fourths, ALL. We prayed, and we once again held on to hope that he was our child.

The birth mom was holding him when we walked into the hospital room. She handed him over to me to hold. As soon as he was in my arms, tears flowed, and my heart just opened right up. It was love at first sight. How could I not love that little guy with all my heart? He melted my heart right then and there.

We had to stay in Iowa for the next ten days until all the paperwork was finished. Needless to say, that was a crazy week and a half. There was lots of joy. But knowing he could be taken away at any moment, there was also lots of anxiety.

After a two-day stay at the hospital, we took little JD to an extended stay hotel where we waited for the final approval. When we finally did get the call on day ten, we hugged and shed tears of joy. He was truly ours! Our son! James Dean Jobe—affectionately known as *JD*. We strapped him into the car seat and took the twelve-hour journey home in our rented car.

When we walked into our home with JD, I could feel my whole body relax and feel at peace. I think he could feel it too. He knew he was home. We made it! We did it! We are parents to this little precious gift from God. I finally get to be a mom! At forty-five years of age, that is, but hey, that's okay! This has been my journey, and I would not trade it for the world.

No two lives are the same, and no two journeys are the same. Life will always have its twists, its turns, and its challenges; but thank you, Jesus, for remaining by my side. You were there in my darkest hours. In my wondering, you were there. In my brokenness, you were there. In everything, you were there.

He never leaves us or forsakes us ever![13] Here's to *New Life*. And here's to *New Hope*.

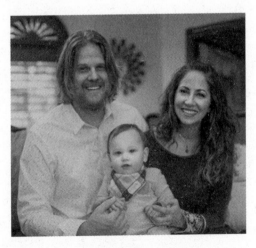

Memarie, Neill, and JD

---

13 "Keep your lives free from the love of money and be content with what you have, because God has said, 'Never will I leave you; never will I forsake you'" (Hebrews 13:5).

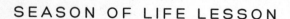

SEASON OF LIFE LESSON

After the first adoption fell through, we were devastated and did not even know if we could push forward to try to adopt again. We took our names off the waiting list for almost two months. I received a message from my pastor a few days after the adoption fell through, and his message simply said, "What Satan means for evil, God will use for good."

I knew that to be true, and I held on to those words. I am so thankful to God that He did not let us give up on adopting the child He had for us. God knew JD before he was even born to this earth, and He knew how perfectly he would fit into our family. JD is the child God gave to us!

We thank you, God, for being faithful in giving us the desires of our hearts.

But as for you, ye thought evil against me; but God meant it unto good, to bring to pass, as it is this day, to save much people alive.
(Genesis 50:20 KJV)

Take delight in the Lord, and he will give you the desires of your heart.
(Psalms 37:4)

You can find the song, *Earth Maker*, on iTunes or Spotify under *Memarie Gayle*.

CHAPTER 12

My Christmas Miracle

My life's journey, like most, has included the highest of highs and the lowest of lows—joy and grief, serenity and discontent, rebellion and surrender, tranquility and turmoil, hope and hopelessness. Through it all, Jesus has been right there with me. At times He was in pursuit of me. Sometimes He picked me up and carried me through. At other times He just walked along beside me and encouraged me to keep going.

But finally, I allowed Him to completely lead me as I followed His will for my life.

This book would not be complete without including my own personal Christmas miracle. I had completed my book, or so I thought, right before I went in for my routine cancer checkup.

I saved it on my computer and set it aside until I could find an editor.

When I received the results from my checkup, I was shocked to find out my CA125 blood marker had gone up for the first time since overcoming cancer in 2014. My stomach dropped, and a flood of emotions came over me.

My oncologist decided to wait a month and check it again—just in case it was a fluke. The month ticked by slowly as I waited for another blood test. The jump in CA125 in the first test was 45. And then the second test showed another jump. At that point a CT scan was ordered.

The CT scan showed no visible cancer, so I was relieved and overjoyed, but I was not in the clear quite yet. My oncologist waited another month and checked my blood again, which test showed a drastic jump to 105. I was devastated! The previous two months had been such a roller coaster ride.

She then ordered a PET scan to look into it further. The days of waiting for the results of the PET scan felt like an eternity. When the call finally came, I heard the voice of my oncologist, who told me it wasn't good news. The only time she personally called me was to tell me the hard-hitting news.

A golf-ball-size mass was seen in my lower right pelvic area, and several lymph nodes were involved as well. "How can this be happening?" I thought.

I felt like I was slowly falling into a black hole of emotion. On the outside I held it together, but on the inside I was fighting a major spiritual battle of emotions. Because of where the mass was sitting, laparoscopic biopsy would need to be performed. The mass was behind my bowel, and to biopsy the mass, there was too great a risk they would puncture my bowel without using laparoscopic tools.

The Thanksgiving holiday was coming up soon, so my doctor decided we could schedule surgery the week after Thanksgiving. Of course that meant another waiting game. The next day was hard to get through without crying. I was home with JD, and I had to walk into my bedroom many times that day so he would not see his mama crying.

Satan was attacking my mind with a vengeance. I rebuked the thoughts and prayed them away, but they kept coming back. I begged and pleaded with God for a healing. I had to be here to see my boy grow up!

"He needs his mama," I pleaded!

For days, as I rocked JD to sleep, I cried in the dark of his nursery, praying in my spirit for a healing. Satan put thoughts of my funeral in my mind, and I rebuked them. He put in my mind thoughts of Neill raising JD alone, and I rebuked them. It was a spiritual battle of the mind, and every moment was a fight to keep my head above water.

On an especially difficult, emotional day, I called my Senior Pastor's wife for prayer. I asked her for two things. I needed her to stand in faith with me that God was healing me, and I needed prayer that my faith would rise up in a big way to meet the healing He had for me. I knew it was God's will to heal me, but I needed my faith to rise up like never before.

After praying for me over the phone, she suggested I have Pastor Sandy anoint me at the first chance I had. It was already late in the week, so I decided to do that Sunday morning after the first service. I began bathing myself in healing Scripture, and instead of reading about ovarian cancer recurrences, I read Scripture.

For days leading up to Sunday I began thanking God for the healing He was already doing in my body. I had healing verses that I highlighted and read aloud every day leading up to that Sunday. When I walked into church, I could still feel a heavy cloud hanging over my head.

I was rebuking the thoughts, I was reading healing Scriptures, but the cloud was still there. It was a constant battle. As I stood on the platform singing in the choir I cried out to God, and I sang His praises—all the while praying that my faith would rise up to meet His healing.

After the service I saw Pastor Sandy step up to the altar benches with the other pastors as they always do in case anyone needs prayer. I quickly went up to her and told her about my latest PET scan showing the tumor in my right pelvic area and the involved lymph nodes. I also told her that Pastor's wife, Gail, told me to have her anoint me. She immediately grabbed the anointing oil from under the altar, anointed my forehead, and began to pray for healing.

I lifted my left hand as I cried out to Jesus and placed my right hand on the area where the tumor was, and Pastor Sandy placed her hand on top of mine. In that moment I felt the power of the all-mighty God like never before. My stomach began to tremble as if an earthquake was happening in my abdomen. It was a vibration that came up through my stomach and back down my legs.

At that moment I was not able to stand, and I fell to the ground trembling and sobbing. The power I felt was overwhelming in that moment. After crying for a bit on the floor I began to laugh, and joy came over my entire being. I knew God had reached down into me with the same power that raised Jesus from the dead, and He had healed me in that moment.

It was like a light switch had flipped on. My faith rose up to meet His healing, and I grabbed it will all my might! Praise Jesus, I knew I had been healed. How did I know? I just knew. When you experience the power of God in that way it is something that words can't describe. I knew in that moment that I had been touched by the power of Jesus, and I physically felt His power manifested within me.

I hugged Pastor Sandy and cried and laughed with joy. I then immediately went to the restroom to be alone with God. I wanted to stay in His close presence as long as I could. I dropped to my knees and cried and thanked Him for what He had done for me. I cried out to Him, and in that moment, He answered me.

I have heard stories of other healings when people didn't feel anything at the moment hands were laid on them, but they were still healed of their illnesses. But God knew I needed a supernatural experience with Him that day, and my faith needed to rise up to meet the healing He already had for me. See, God wants to heal us! We just have to reach deep inside ourselves and let our faith rise up to meet His healing.

This is easier said than done because Satan can promote to us lots of lies. The lies can come through doctors, symptoms, statistics, negative thoughts, circumstances—you name it, he uses it. But God is much bigger than all of this! God is bigger than cancer, bigger than any disease, and bigger than any affliction you might have.

Some people teach others to deny their problems and simply not accept them. But that's not the solution. Before being healed by God—before placing yourself in the position of reaching up to receive what you need from God—you must fully acknowledge your need and then accept His solution. You don't deny that you have a problem, you simply first believe that God can heal you, and then you have to reach out to Him for the healing.

You have to activate your faith. You do this by reading and listening to the Word, by speaking God's promises out loud, by letting them sink into your spirit, and by putting them into action. When I left church that Sunday, I walked out like a different person from the one who walked in.

The light switch of faith was on, and it was shining brightly. I didn't have to try to be joyful; I was joyful, and I knew beyond a doubt that God healed me. I didn't know if I had received an instant healing, a gradual healing, or a healing that I would have to walk through and allow Him to work through others for me to realize, but I knew God's healing virtue had been placed inside me.

During that time, we were in heavy rehearsals for a large Christmas production at my church, and we had been rehearsing for months. It was going to be the largest production we had done in the history of our church. I had two solos and was in several choir ensembles. I was determined that I was not going to bow out, and I really felt I would be blessed through being in it.

I have found that when I use the gifts God has given me, He always sends blessings my way. I also knew that in order for me to appear in the production, I had to delay my laparoscopic surgery for another week—making it three weeks past the time I received my PET scan results. I looked at my participation in the Christmas program as me putting my faith into action. I verbally spoke it to others, and I was determined to put it into action by going ahead with my part.

I held on to my healing and renewed faith with all I had in me, but it didn't come easily. For the first week after my healing I was on a spiritual high, looking up everything I could about healing in the Scriptures. I also looked up other people's testimonies on healing.

During that time, I had been taking several anti-cancer herbs that I had purchased from an herbalist. One night while making up my nightly concoction of herbs, I accidently put a teaspoon of hydrogen peroxide in my cup with my portioned-out herbs. The herbalist had put a high-graded hydrogen peroxide in a glass bottle that looked just like my herbs.

I was only supposed to put a drop of hydrogen peroxide in a 16-ounce container of water. I was a little leery of it, so I wasn't even using it for that, but it was sitting next to all my other herbs. As soon as I threw back my concoction of herbs, I knew something was wrong, and I immediately knew I had ingested hydrogen peroxide because I could feel it bubbling in my throat. It felt like my throat was starting to close.

My Mom was sitting on the couch when that happened, so I yelled for her to call 911. Neill and JD were on the porch and didn't realize what was going on. Instinctively I ran to the kitchen and started downing bottled waters. I probably drank at least four bottles. Mom ran out to get Neill, and she stayed with JD as he rushed me to the emergency room.

I was terrified! I threw up all the way to the hospital, and by the time I got there the bloating in my stomach had gone down, and I was feeling much better. But the doctor opted to keep me overnight for observation to be safe. Apparently, such a thing could cause a heart attack, stroke, or worse.

They ran many tests, which all came back fine. They said all the water I drank immediately after ingesting the hydrogen peroxide saved me and caused me to throw it up fairly quickly. I was so angry at myself. Jesus touched me with His healing power, and less than a week later I ingest hydrogen peroxide. I could not believe I had done something so extremely stupid!

I was so disappointed in myself. But on top of it all, Satan used that to get me back in a worrying state of mind. I began worrying that I had possibly damaged my heart. After all, the doctor in the ER said that was possible. And on top of all that, I still had symptoms in my lower pelvic area.

Then Satan had a small win over the Thanksgiving holiday, but in the end, Jesus had the victory—as He always does!

We went to Orange Beach, Alabama, as is our tradition, to spend Thanksgiving with Neill's family. Each year they rent a condo, and our entire family goes for the week and has a big Thanksgiving dinner there with our beach-front view. A couple of nights before Thanksgiving I was sitting on the couch with the family, and my chest was feeling tight. I was getting little twinges of pain and felt like I needed to take deep breaths.

Neill looked over at me, and I was evidently as white as a ghost. He asked me if I was okay, and in that moment, I started feeling super cold and lightheaded. I told him I didn't feel right, and I was having chest pains. About that time my hands started to feel tingly and numb. The family immediately called the ER because I thought I was having a heart attack. In my mind the hydrogen peroxide incident had damaged my heart, and it was coming back to haunt me.

Once the ambulance got there the EMT's checked me out and said my heart seemed fine, but they thought I should go to the ER and have more tests run. That was a nightmare! There I was going to an ER for the second time in one week.

Once I got to the ER my symptoms had lessened but were not totally gone. After running all their tests, the doctor concluded that I had an anxiety attack. But that was like no anxiety attack I had before. I felt physical pain in my chest, chills, and tingly hands. But I was informed that all of those things can be brought on by anxiety. Once I knew that, I knew how to fight it. I fought it with Scripture, and I rebuked it in Jesus' name.

Once I knew my heart was fine, I was able to get out of my funk and get back to the peace God had for me. That was just a wrench Satan had thrown into the mix to keep me from the peace and joy of God. I threw myself into Scripture like never before, and I continued thanking God for my healing He had given me that Sunday on the second of December, 2018.

I made a decision in the ER that Satan was not going to taunt me anymore! I called the anxiety out by name, and I commanded it to leave in Jesus' name. No stupid hydrogen peroxide accident was going to keep me from my healing. God was bigger than all of it! The closer we get to something great and wonderful that God has for us the harder Satan fights to keep us from it.

After that anxiety attack, I knew it was an attack by Satan himself, and I was not having it. That would not be his last effort, but that *would be* his last win!

After returning home to Nashville from our Thanksgiving on the beach, I jumped back into our church Christmas production rehearsals. That was my chance to walk out my faith and use my gifts to bring more people into the kingdom. We did three performances, and it was such a blessing to be a part of each one.

Singing praises to God the entire week leading up to my laparoscopic surgery was the best thing I could have done to prepare myself. I felt strong both physically, mentally, and emotionally when I went into surgery. As my doctor stood in my pre-op room going through the procedure, I took it all in with a grain of salt, because I was standing on faith that I was healed.

No scans had been performed since I was anointed and prayed for at church. And going into the operating room, I had a peace that God was going to be revealed that day. As I was laying there waiting for them to give me the anesthesia, the nurse asked me if I would like to hear any music to relax by? She opened the computer in the room, and I had her go to an online praise and worship station.

The first song to come on was the Lauren Daigle song, *Oh Lord*—the song that I listened to every day throughout my cancer fight four years earlier. It always lifted my spirits. The choice of that song was no coincidence. As I thanked God for that joyful song, I drifted off to sleep.

When I woke up from surgery I was greeted by my oncologist with a bewildered look on her face. She proceeded to tell me that the tumor was gone, and all my lymph nodes looked normal.

I could not contain myself as I threw my hands up crying out, "Thank you Jesus. Thank you Jesus!"

I told her God had healed me, and He was taking care of me. She was in what looked like shock as she told me she had two other oncologists come into the operating room to double check her findings.

That was my Christmas miracle. Thank you, Father God. You are always faithful.

EPILOGUE

I believe the *soul* is the core of who we are. It's the part of us that makes us all unique individuals. It's the part where God puts His signature on us—for His purpose in our lives. And it is up to us to find that purpose and to live it out.

If we have asked Jesus to come into our hearts—if we have turned our lives over to Him—then He is living within us. Our spirits are one with Him, and every day He is molding our bodies and our souls to come into complete alignment with His spirit.

I believe we should always be reaching for the *higher self* that God is attempting to mold us into. Our wonderful creator's fingerprint is on each and every one of us. If you are still searching for your purpose, simply ask God to use His Holy Spirit to help guide you to that purpose. God is always faithful, so I have no doubt that your purpose will be revealed.

I encourage you to put a pen and paper, or even a small recorder, beside your bed, because when you are diligently praying for an answer from God, He will sometimes give you a word in the middle of the night. Even if you're not sure the thoughts that come to you in the night are from God, just write them down and meditate on them in the morning.

While writing this book I woke up early one morning from a dream with an image in my head and the words, "Journey Back to the Soul" written above it. I immediately grabbed a pen and paper, drew it out, and saved it. The image reflects the pathway I took while journeying back to my soul.

God recently revealed to me that the image was a fingerprint—His fingerprint on my life. For my *next* forty-seven years, I pray that I will grow closer and closer to Christ with each passing day—therefore, closer and closer to the person He created me to be.

I don't know where my life's journey will lead me from here, but I do know God will be by my side as He always is. And I know the same healing power that brought to me my Christmas miracle in 2018 will continue to be manifested in my body for complete restoration of health.

So now, another journey begins.

You can find my song, *Soul Time*, on iTunes or
Spotify under *Memarie Gayle.*

JOURNEY BACK TO THE SOUL

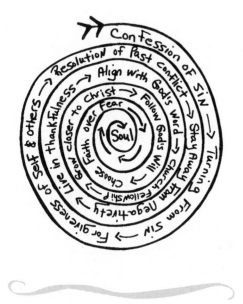

If you have not yet given your life over to God, I encourage you to pray this prayer out loud to God, now.

> God, I confess my sins to you now and ask for your gracious forgiveness. I believe that you sent your Son, Jesus Christ, to earth to die on the cross for my sins. I accept Him in my heart now as my Lord and Savior. Please send your Holy Spirit to lead and guide me to do your will in my life from this day forward.
>
> In Jesus' name, Amen.

ABOUT THE AUTHOR

Memarie Gayle Jobe lives in Nashville, Tennessee, with her husband, Neill, their son, JD, their two cats, Betty and Boop, and their dog, Snickers. Memarie is the owner/lead designer of *Fearless Memories Jewelry*. She continues her musical passion through writing and recording songs and singing on the praise and worship team at Cornerstone Nashville Church.

In her *Faith Over Fear* ministry, Memarie visits abuse shelters, conducts jewelry workshops, and shares her testimony. She also speaks and sings at churches, conferences, and retreats.

Memarie serves on the organizing committee of *Chic Awearness*, a Nashville-based organization that raises funds for ovarian cancer research. Chicawearness.org

Memarie collaborated with fellow ovarian cancer survivor, Leora Allen, to design the *Power of Awareness* jewelry collection to bring awareness to the early signs and symptoms of ovarian cancer.

She also organized the event, *Songs for Cancer*, in honor of her late father, Jerry Cupit. The event held in Nashville every other year has raised thousands of dollars for Myelofibrosis Research at Vanderbilt Ingram Cancer Center.

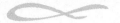

To learn more about Memarie, her philanthropy
efforts, music, and handcrafted jewelry,
visit Fearlessmemories.com

Find Memarie Gayle's music on *iTunes* and *Spotify*.

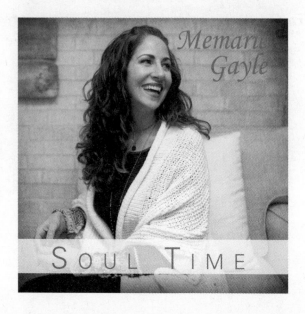

Instructions for receiving your free music album:

1. Send an e-mail message to:
   jouneybacktothesoul@bridgelogos.com
   and request your copy of the album.

2. Include the following in your message:
   - Your Full Name
   - Your Full Address
   - The Date you purchased *Journey Back to the Soul*
   - Where you purchased the book (the name and location of the Physical Store, Event, or Online Retail Outlet)

3. In return, you will receive by e-mail a special single-use code with instructions on how to download your free copy of Memarie Gayle's new album.

This offer may expire or be withdrawn without notice
if the book is out-of-print or the offer is no longer
included in future printings.

BEAUTY FROM ASHES
Donna Sparks

In a transparent and powerful manner, the author reveals how the Lord took her from the ashes of a life devastated by failed relationships and destructive behavior to bring her into a beautiful and powerful relationship with Him. The author encourages others to allow the Lord to do the same for them.

Donna Sparks is an Assemblies of God evangelist who travels widely to speak at women's conferences and retreats. She lives in Tennessee.

www.story-of-grace.com

www.facebook.com/
donnasparksministries/

www.facebook.com/
AuthorDonnaSparks/

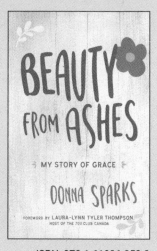

ISBN: 978-1-61036-252-8

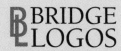

BRIDGE
LOGOS